TRICIA YU

tai chi
mind and body

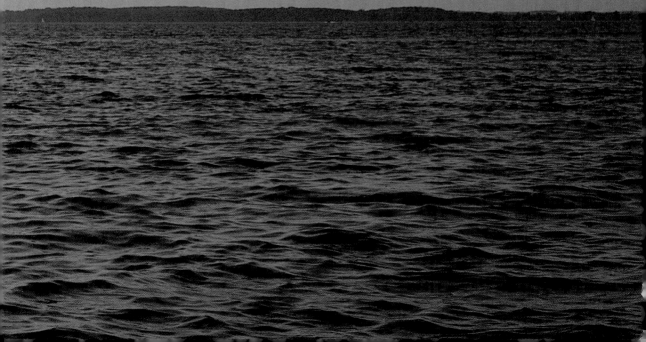

LONDON, NEW YORK, MELBOURNE,
MUNICH and DELHI

To Clarissa, Dayton, Maggie, Roscoe, Aidan and Owen

Project Editor Nasim Mawji
Art Editor Bill Mason
Senior Editor Jennifer Jones
Managing Editor Gillian Roberts
Art Director Tracy Killick
Category Publisher Mary-Clare Jerram
DTP Designer Sonia Charbonnier
Picture researcher Suzanne Bosman
Production Controller Joanna Bull

First published in Great Britain in 2003
by Dorling Kindersley Limited
80 Strand, London WC2R 0RL
Penguin Group (UK)

A CIP catalogue record for this book is available
from The British Library

ISBN 0 7513 6449 5

Colour reproduced in Singapore by Colourscan
Printed and bound by MOHN Media and
Mohndruck GmbH, Germany

CONTENTS

  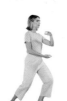 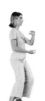 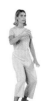

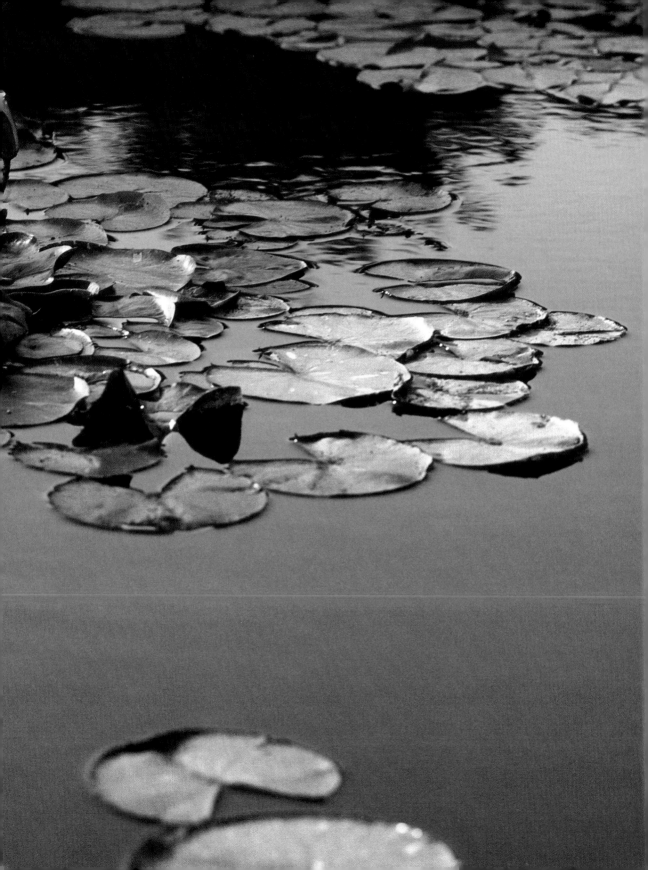

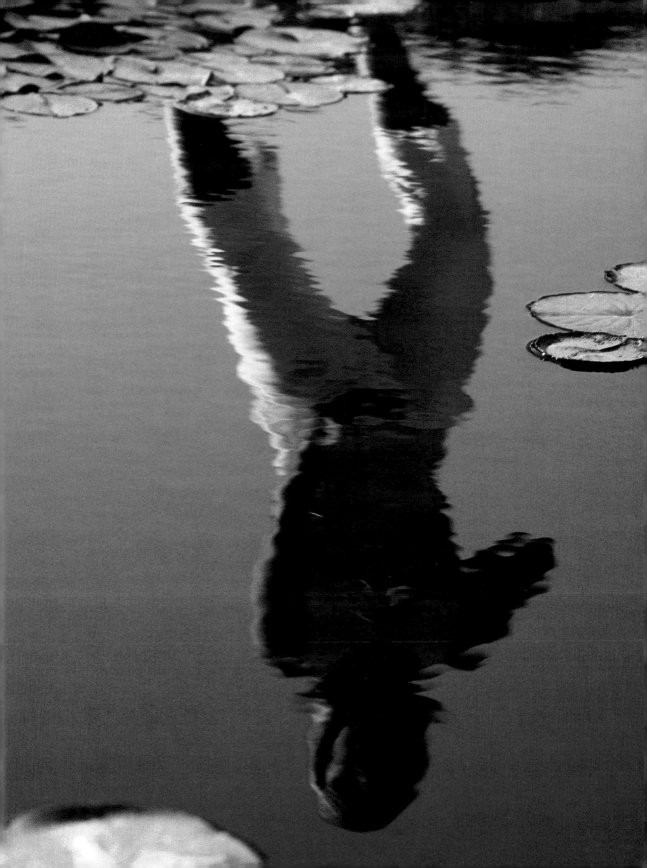

WHAT IS TAI CHI?

Tai chi, also known as *tai chi ch'uan*, is an ancient Chinese exercise that combines relaxed, fluid movement with a calm, alert mental state. It looks like an effortless, slow-motion dance. Developed more than 700 years ago by Chinese martial artists, it is a non-impact exercise that builds endurance and enhances flexibility, balance, and coordination. Growing numbers of people worldwide are finding that this combination of movement and mental focus constitutes an excellent fitness regime for both mind and body.

Tai chi translates from Chinese as "supreme ultimate": the centre of things or the common source that unifies all apparent opposites. Tai chi ch'uan (also written "Taiji" or "Taijiquan") means "supreme ultimate boxing or fist". It applies the principle of staying centred, both mentally and physically, in the midst of conflict.

I first encountered tai chi in 1969 when my husband and I had just moved to Taiwan. Early one morning, I came across a park filled with hundreds of people doing slow, graceful exercises. To my surprise, the elderly moved with the balance and fluidity of the young, executing low squats, high kicks, and spins on one leg

with apparently no exertion. Some of these people looked like they were in their 80s, and yet they were fit. My curiosity was aroused, and over a year later, I was accepted as the only non-Chinese student of Liu Pei Ch'ung, a famous Taoist master. Since then I have continued daily practice of tai chi for what is now well over thirty years.

I remember three distinct, seemingly contradictory experiences when I first began learning tai chi. First of all, it felt remarkably calm and peaceful moving slowly and quietly with a group of other people. At the same time, I became acutely aware of the tension I had held in my body and the distractions in my mind. Finally, it felt energizing — a novel sort of awake and alive feeling.

THE BENEFITS OF TAI CHI

Tai chi can be practised by people of all ages and most physical conditions. Regular practice helps develop healthy breathing patterns and relaxation skills. As a non-impact exercise it strengthens the body with minimal stress to the joints. In addition, it improves body awareness, postural alignment, coordination, strength,

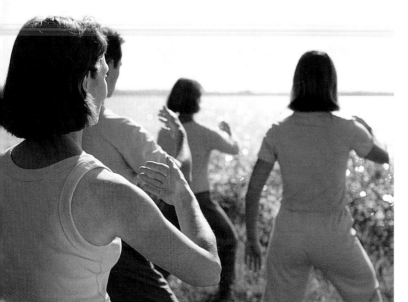

A tranquil lake provides an inspirational setting for tai chi practice. Consider the stillness of a clear pool and the power of a waterfall. Keep your movements fluid.

In China I have seen tai chi practised everywhere – between parked cars by busy streets, even in train stations and airports. Here, I teach tai chi on a city rooftop terrace.

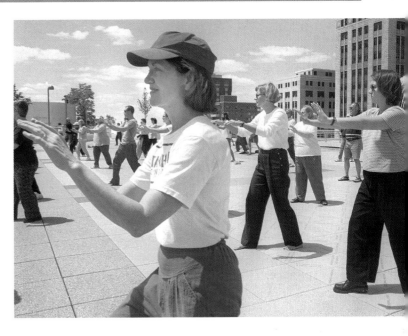

and flexibility. Tai chi trains you to relax your external muscles and utilize deeper structural muscles, which strengthens the tendons and the bones. When I first began tai chi, what surprised me was the workout on my legs – the seemingly effortless grace of the movements is deceptive. Tai chi trains proper body alignment as you move; it teaches you to take the stress off the back, hips, and shoulders, and to allow the large muscles in the legs to support your weight.

It is a moderately aerobic exercise that can reduce stress levels and enhance the body's immune response. Regular practice lowers blood pressure and promotes emotional well-being. It is also an ideal weight-bearing exercise that helps improve balance.

Finally, tai chi teaches you to move with effortless grace, a skill that can be applied to any activity from running, wind surfing, rock climbing, and basketball to walking, lifting objects, and even playing a musical instrument. This ancient Chinese "supreme ultimate" exercise has universal applications.

THE ORIGINS OF TAI CHI

Tai chi originated in China around the 13th century AD as a synthesis of martial arts exercise and sitting meditation. Its legendary founder, Chang San Feng, inspired by a graceful crane and supple coiling snake in battle, devised an evolved system of self-defence based not on brute strength and physical force but on the power of flow and flexibility, yielding, rooting and returning energy. In addition to its martial arts benefits, tai chi was practised for cultivating healthy flow of vital energy, or qi (see p20).

RECENT HISTORY

For many centuries, tai chi was practised secretly, passed on from father to son in the Chen Village in northern China. In the mid-1800s Master Yang Lu Shan became the first outsider to learn tai chi, and as the commander of the imperial guards taught this advanced self-defence method to his men. It soon became popular in martial arts circles and branched into three main styles, each named after its founder (Yang, Chen, and Wu).

In the early 20th century Lu Shan's grandson, Master Yang Cheng Fu, modified his family's form; then, in the 1930s, his famous student Cheng Man Ch'ing shortened and simplified the form in order to make it accessible as a health exercise, while maintaining its martial arts applications. Since then, tai chi has enjoyed widespread popularity in China.

In the late sixties, tai chi began to take root in the United States and Europe. Grand Master Cheng Man Ch'ing came to New York where he opened a large tai chi school, and was one of the first to teach tai chi openly to non-Chinese students. Since then, Masters Benjamin Pang Jeng Lo and William C.C. Chen and other students of Cheng Man Ch'ing's have taught tai chi to thousands of students across the United States and Europe, making this version of Yang-Style tai chi one of the most popular forms worldwide.

THE FUNDAMENTALS PROGRAMME

Tai chi remains elusive to many who find its complex movements confusing and difficult to master, and the terminology and concepts hard to grasp. I created the Tai Chi Fundamentals Programme presented in this book to help address this issue. The programme offers a clear system for mastering the basics of tai chi while still retaining the integrity of the traditional Yang-Style form and the mind–body principles. It simplifies moves that students consistently find difficult when learning tai chi but still includes critical elements from the traditional form that enhance balance, coordination, strength, and endurance. The programme provides a good groundwork for learning or refining your tai chi practice.

THE MIND–BODY CONNECTION

Like yoga, tai chi originated in a culture that views the mind and body not as separate but rather as different expressions or states of qi – vital energy or life force.

According to ancient Chinese medicine, our thoughts and emotions have a direct effect on our physical health. In addition, the climate, the seasons, and the weather – external factors – affect our health. Everything influences the qi that flows through the meridians, or channels, within the body. The ancient Chinese medical model mapped the effects of different emotional states on health. For example, too much anger is believed to harm the liver, too much sadness the spleen, and too much fear the kidneys. Illness is thought to be an indication of imbalance within the body as well as between the body and the environment. Harmony and balance are believed to bring about good health and well-being.

THE TAO OF TAI CHI

The Taoist perspective was integral to the philosophy and culture of China for thousands of years and naturally influenced the development of tai chi. "Tao" means "road" or "path" for living a simple, peaceful life in harmony with the natural world. Taoists believe that all elements of the universe are interconnected. This is worth reflecting upon as you practise tai chi. The same concept is illustrated in the tai chi diagram, or yin–yang symbol:

The outer circle symbolizes unity – or Wu Chi – that is, all that exists is contained within the same whole, and there is infinite potential for variety. All of our inner experiences, such as feelings, emotions, and sensations, as well as those that are external, such as other people, the natural world, the planets, and stars are all simply different expressions of the same whole. We are all one.

The dark and light areas of the symbol indicate that within the unity, we perceive duality. For example, male/female, me/you, dark/light, right/wrong, in/out. There is so much variety in our world that we identify things by their differences rather than inherent sameness.

The small circles within the dark and light areas represent the fact that, although we perceive ourselves from the perspective of our separateness, there is nothing that is entirely separate from anything else.

The centre of the symbol represents the balance point for all aspects of life. This is the still point that unifies all apparent opposites. As we shift our perspective more to the centre of any situation we take a fundamental step in the cultivation of tai chi mind – the middle way, the path of peace.

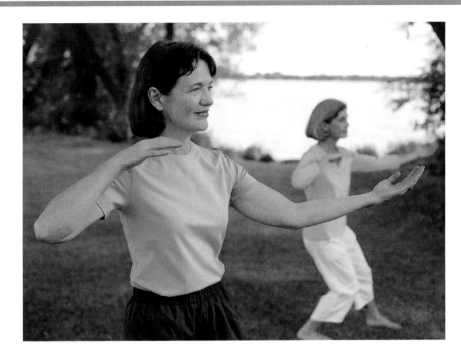

Tai chi practice can have a beneficial effect on your mental and emotional states, as well as help you to feel connected with your surroundings.

In the West, the mind and body have been traditionally viewed as separate. However, as methods of research and technology become more sophisticated, science is beginning to acknowledge the mind–body connection. As Deepak Chopra MD wrote, "invisible wisps of thought and emotion alter the fundamental chemistry of every cell."

Countless factors influence our health, but research has shown that our mental states can affect us physically. For example, a calm, quiet state of mind and a sense of emotional well-being actually reduce levels of cortisol, which the body produces when it is stressed. Similarly, a peaceful feeling and self-acceptance enhance the immune response by raising the T-cell count. Research has also shown that active participation and experiencing a sense of relationship to others and to one's source of spiritual inspiration can have a beneficial effect on the body. All of these mental states actually help to keep you healthy.

On the other hand, feeling chronically stressed, overworked or overwhelmed, depressed, anxious, hopeless, fearful, and worried can suppress immune function. In addition, loneliness, fear of change, lack of control, and feeling powerless all contribute to lowered resiliency levels in the body.

Our inner life, our thoughts, attitudes, and emotions all influence our health. Practising tai chi, especially outside in natural surroundings, can have a beneficial effect on your mental and emotional states as well as help you to feel connected with the world around you.

TAI CHI MIND

Regular practice of tai chi helps you to focus your mind without forming rigid attachment to a single point of view. This is known as tai chi mind: perceiving the unifying elements of a situation rather than those that divide, and remembering that there is always an element within you of that which you oppose. This perspective on life encourages harmony and a sense of connection. It is the best state of mind for dealing with fearful or stressful situations or with conflict, confusion, or disappointment. It teaches you to focus, to move from the eye of the hurricane and not be swept away in the surrounding confusion.

CENTRING

Tai chi practice generally begins with a few moments of quiet while focusing on slow, natural breathing to help calm the mind, relax the body, and bring attention into the present moment. Known as "centring", this process is rarely included in Western forms of exercise and has valuable applications beyond tai chi. Learning to relax and quiet your mind helps you to connect with other people and your surroundings, and to feel more responsive to what is occurring around you.

Many of us lead hectic and stressful lives, and it is easy to become absorbed by worries about the future, or events of the past – sometimes to the extent that we don't notice what is actually occurring in the present. According to the principles of tai chi, this depletes your qi. Being aware of the present moment, in touch with your body's signals, more sensitive to others and to your surroundings enhances your qi.

Ideally, practise centring alone and in silence or with quiet, calming background music. Watching television or listening to loud music will distract you and disconnect the mind from the body.

Once you learn to focus your attention, you can integrate this exercise into empty moments in your day: waiting in line, on hold, at traffic lights, at your computer, or on the train or underground, for example.

How to centre

You can practise this exercise sitting, standing, or lying down. Use it as an effective stress-reduction technique, even when walking. Find a quiet, comfortable place outside in the fresh air, if possible. You can have your eyes open or closed. Take as little as a few seconds, or as long as several minutes.

- **Bring your attention** into the present moment.
- **Notice your breathing,** and feel the movement in your body as you inhale and exhale.
- **Relax.**
- **Notice the position of your body**. Keep your body upright and naturally aligned.
- **Bring your awareness** into your hands and fingers, then into your feet and head.
- **Relax as you focus** on your breathing, head, hands, and feet.
- **Notice** the different sounds, sights, and smells that surround you.

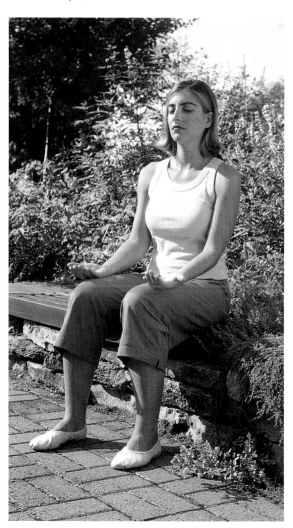

Centring helps you to focus mentally, which is essential for tai chi and a key ingredient for health of body and mind.

TAI CHI MOVEMENT PRINCIPLES

Keep these guidelines in mind as you embark upon your tai chi practice. They will enhance your experience of tai chi and help to make it as rewarding and fulfilling as possible. Remember that tai chi principles can be applied to all activity, not just tai chi.

Focus

Bring your attention into the present while maintaining awareness of your body and your surroundings. Concentrate on each precise movement, your breathing, and the position of your body. Tai chi trains you to combine mental focus and physical action. This skill develops gradually as a result of regular practice.

Relax actively

This may sound contradictory, but this state actually enables you to perform at your best. It means achieving a state of relaxed inner stillness while in motion. This state requires minimal use of the muscles while also maintaining a relaxed awareness of the whole body.

Maintain a natural posture

Keep your body upright with your head erect, back straight, shoulders aligned over your hips, and feet flat.

Notice your breathing

Breathe naturally through your nose. Relax your belly so that it expands as you inhale and contracts as you exhale. Avoid holding your breath while concentrating — maintain a regular breathing pattern (*see pp18–19*).

Move slowly

Most exercise programmes focus on exertion and straining as a means to achieving increased strength and endurance. In contrast, tai chi builds strength and endurance through slow, relaxed, continuous movement in a flexed stance. The slower and lower the movement, the greater the strength and endurance benefit.

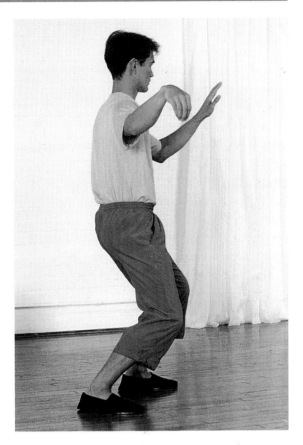

Aim to move naturally and effectively and to keep your body properly aligned. Remain balanced and focused, and be aware of your breathing at all times.

Separate your weight

Balancing entirely on one foot is known as "separating the weight" — it helps establish balance and dramatically increases leg strength. During transitions and when shifting weight, keep your body upright and make sure that 100 percent of your weight rests on your stable foot.

Move from your centre

Consider the head, torso, and pelvis as a single "column" aligned over the stable base in your legs and feet. All arm and hand movements are initiated by the upright rotation of this "column". There is no twisting of the spine. Also called "core movement", it creates the effortless-looking flow of motion characteristic of tai chi.

GETTING STARTED

Tai chi is more than a fitness routine; it is an exercise for lifelong well-being. Keep up any other exercise that you do, and simply add tai chi to your regime. You can do it almost anywhere, at any time. It requires no special equipment, and a practice session need take only a few minutes a day.

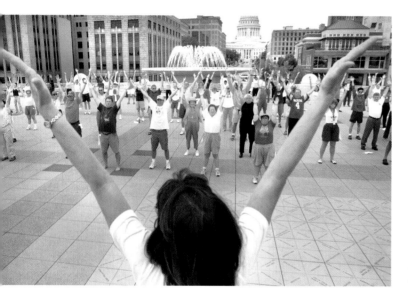

Tai chi has universal appeal, regardless of your age or fitness level. It helps you to feel both relaxed and energized.

HOW TO USE THIS BOOK

This book will be useful to beginners as well as advanced practitioners and tai chi instructors. For greatest benefit, avoid rushing through it. Tai chi is a slow, meditative exercise; take a calm and thoughtful approach to learning it.

The Basic Moves and the Form are presented in three corresponding parts. Each part builds on the previous one and progresses in difficulty. Begin by practicing Part One of the Basic Moves, repeating each move several times with focus on your alignment, footwork, and flow of qi. Learn each move by heart before proceeding to the next. When you are confident with your technique in each of the Basic Moves in a part, proceed to the corresponding part in the Form. The Form integrates the moves into a flowing sequence of

tai chi. As you practise the Form, refer back to the Basic Moves to check your technique is correct.

A unique feature of this book is the floor grid in the Basic Moves and the Form. It is four squares across by three squares deep; each square is roughly hip-width. In this book, each square was 30 cm (1 ft) square. The grid will help you position your feet correctly during a tai chi sequence. It may help to practise on a tiled floor or on floorboards, or create your own grid to help establish your stances properly.

HOW AND WHERE TO PRACTISE

Initially, try practising in front of a full-length mirror so that you can check your posture. Or team up with a friend so that you can give each other feedback. If you practise daily for 15 minutes, allow at least one week to learn each part of the Basic Moves, and one week for each part of the Form. It will take at least six weeks, and probably longer, to learn all of the moves.

Once you have learned the moves, you can practise almost anywhere, but if possible practise outside in the fresh air — in your garden, on the beach, or in a quiet park. At first you may feel uneasy practising outside, but as you establish a routine, you will feel more comfortable.

WHEN TO PRACTISE

Tai chi is a wonderful way to start the day. I always practise in the morning after a cup of tea and before breakfast. If you practise at other times, remember to wait one hour after eating. The entire programme takes about 20 minutes to complete, but you can easily devise a shorter routine by practising just one or two moves. A session can take as long as 45 minutes or as little as 3 minutes. The important thing is just to do a little each day. This will be easier if you establish a regular time and place for practice. Regardless of the length of your session, always try to include the following in your routine:

- **Begin** with at least one or two minutes of centring (*see p12*) to calm your mind and relax your body.
- **Follow** with the warm-up exercises (*see pp24–29*), which take about three minutes to complete.
- **Work through the Basic Moves** and then the Form as suggested, or pick just one or two moves to practise. If there is less time, do fewer moves—it is counterproductive to rush through them.
- **You can also practise** holding the positions for several seconds initially and eventually for up to one minute or more.
- **Pause for a minute or so** of quiet contemplation at the end of your session. You can also practise the standing exercises for sensing qi (*see pp22–23*), or the qi exercises in the Subtle Energy of Tai Chi (*see pp146–153*).

WHAT TO WEAR

You do not need any special clothing or footwear in order to practise tai chi. Wear anything designed for exercise, or loose, comfortable clothing that allows you to breathe easily. Wear shoes with low heels, go barefoot, or wear socks. Footwear should leave ample room for your toes. Wear shoes made of a breathable fabric such as cotton, with flexible soles that bend with your feet. Unless you have a condition that requires wearing special support, avoid wearing shoes designed for high-impact workouts, and avoid high-top shoes as they can inhibit ankle movement.

MEDICAL CONSIDERATIONS

Tai chi is a safe and gentle exercise for people of all ages and most physical conditions. When practising, listen to your body's signals; do not attempt any movements that feel in any way uncomfortable, and stop immediately if you experience any pain.

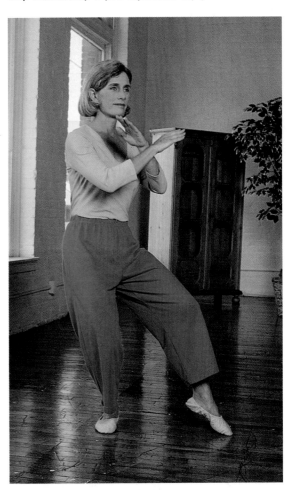

You can practise tai chi almost anywhere. Wear loose, comfortable clothing that allows you to move freely, and simple shoes with flat heels – or go barefoot.

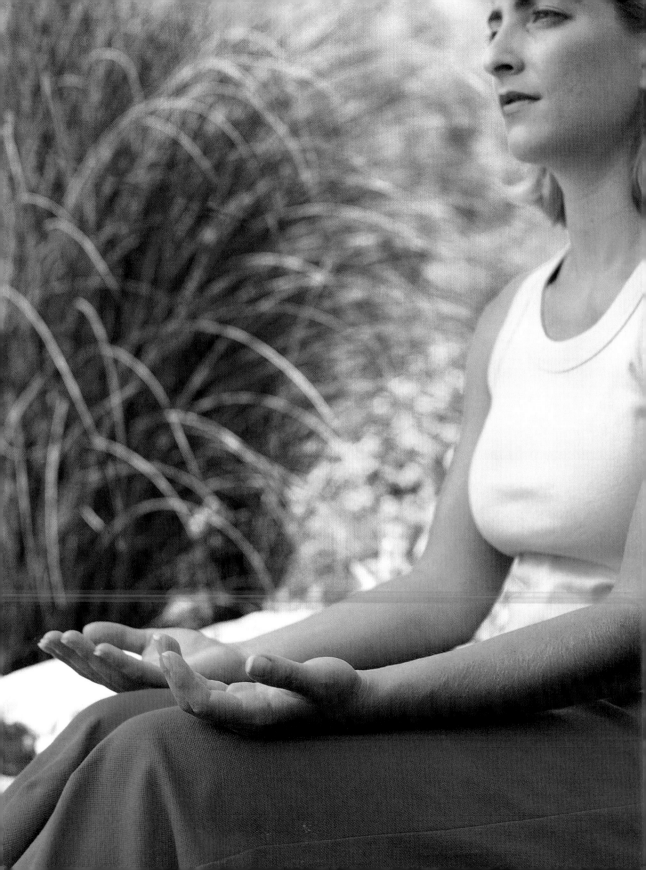

THE
ESSENTIALS
OF
TAI CHI

The pages that follow familiarize you with the three essential elements of tai chi: breathing in a relaxed, natural, and healthy manner; sensing qi (life energy), or becoming more alive to each moment; and warming up slowly and gently so that your movements are fluid and relaxed. Together these essentials have a subtly energizing effect on the body, preparing you, both physically and mentally, for your tai chi practice.

BREATHING

This is where it all begins. Here you learn to focus on your breathing and develop a slow, relaxed breathing pattern. This helps you to achieve the relaxed, alert state of both mind and body that is essential for the practice of tai chi. Breathing naturally and from the diaphragm, or belly breathing, is not just for tai chi practice – it is the healthiest way to breathe at all times.

NATURAL BREATHING

Air provides the basic nourishment for the body. The way that you breathe has a direct effect on the way that you feel. Most adults tend to tense the lower abdomen in order to hold their bellies as flat as possible when they breathe. This prevents the lower portion of the lungs from filling with air, resulting in less oxygen for the body per breath. Known as "chest breathing", this can contribute to a feeling of stress. For many, shallow chest breathing is a habit that feels perfectly normal.

When you inhale naturally, your lungs fill fully with air, which pushes your diaphragm down, causing your belly to expand. As you exhale, your diaphragm moves back up and your belly naturally contracts. This natural, diaphragmatic breathing pattern is known as "belly breathing", and it supplies the body with optimal oxygen per breath.

Natural diaphragmatic breathing promotes what scientists refer to as the "relaxation response", or a reduction of the indicators of stress. It brings about a decrease in blood pressure and heart rate and increases blood flow to the extremities. In addition, people report a general feeling of well-being. Developing natural breathing patterns is one of the most important things you can do for your health.

BREATH AWARENESS

The first step in developing healthy breathing patterns is simply to get in touch with your breathing. Take a few minutes just to feel and observe yourself breathing. Most people find, initially, that lying down is the best position for this (*see below*), but you can practise in any position as long as you are comfortable and your body is well-aligned and supported. Try any of the positions for Belly Breathing (*see opposite*). As you breathe, consider that breath is the thread that connects all living things, and that everything that lives, breathes.

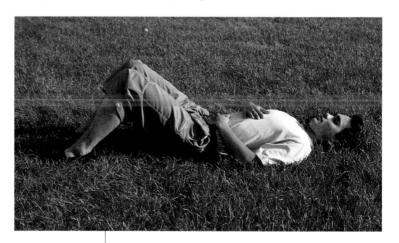

Lie on your back with your hands on your belly and chest so you feel the movement in your body as you breathe. Bend your knees so that your feet are flat; this takes pressure off the lower back.

BELLY BREATHING

When you feel ready, practise breathing deeply and with your diaphragm. As your belly expands and contracts, you are effortlessly strengthening your abdominal muscles. Choose any comfortable position – for example, lying on your back or face down, or sitting (*see opposite and below*). To help feel the movement as you breathe, place one hand on your chest and the other on your belly, or place both hands on your belly.

- **Breathe normally,** and notice where you feel the movement within your body.
- **Relax.** Notice any thoughts, feelings, and physical sensations that you experience.
- **Focus your mind.** As you inhale, think "breathe in", and as you exhale, think "breathe out".
- **Feel your body expanding** as you inhale and contracting as you exhale.
- **Imagine** as you breathe in that your belly is filling up like a balloon, then emptying as you breathe out.
- **Sense your abdominal muscles** actively expanding as you inhale, and contracting as you exhale.

Once you can consistently experience belly breathing in one position, you can apply the principles when sitting, standing, walking, and practising tai chi. Whenever you feel tense, fearful, or worried, simply focus on your breathing to help you relax.

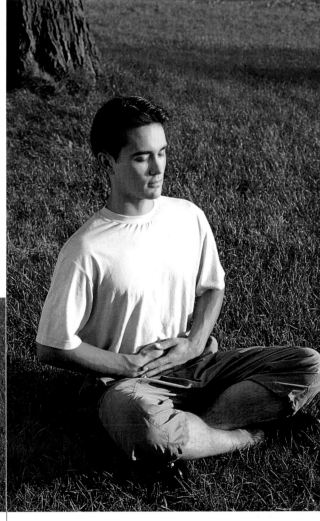

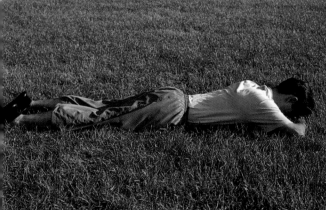

Lie face down with your forehead resting on your hands. As you breathe in, feel your belly push against the ground as gravity helps to expand it. As you breathe out, feel your belly release from the ground.

Sit with your back straight and shoulders relaxed, and place your hands on your belly. It is easier to breathe from the belly when your body is upright and naturally aligned.

SENSING QI

Tai chi is a form of qi cultivation or "qigong". Qi (also spelled ch'i) translates from Chinese as "life energy" or "life force", and gong means "skill". Qi has been acknowledged in many different cultures. The ancient Greeks called it *pneuma*, in India it is called *prana*, and the Japanese refer to it as *ki*. In China, it is an ordinary term and part of the common language; for example, the weather is called *tien qi*, or "heaven qi", and air is called *kung qi*, or "empty qi".

BECOMING AWARE OF QI

A natural setting is the most conducive for feeling qi, but any peaceful, quiet setting, away from external distractions, will do. To develop awareness of qi, you first need to practise bringing your attention into the present and focusing on the moment. You can develop awareness of qi through being quiet and sensing your own body. The simple exercises that follow will help you to develop awareness of qi. They teach you to relax and to focus on your breathing — a good way to heighten awareness of sensation in your body. Begin with the lying position for sensing qi, which allows you to relax more easily, then move on to the sitting and standing positions (*see opposite and pp22–23*). Most people feel

SENSING QI WHILE LYING DOWN

Make sure that you are in a relaxed, comfortable position with your legs uncrossed. You may wish to bend your knees so that your feet are flat on the floor. Spend at least 3–4 minutes or much longer on this exercise.

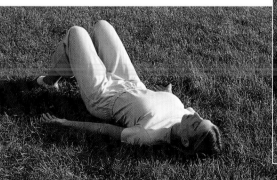

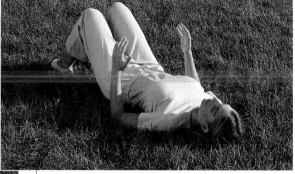

1 Place one hand on your belly and one on your chest and focus on your breathing (*see p18*), then move your hands to your sides, palms facing upwards. Notice any changes in sensation in your hands and fingers as you breathe in and out.

2 Keep your elbows on the floor, and raise your hands so that your palms face each other with fingers pointing upwards, wrists straight and relaxed. Notice the sensation between your hands as you breathe. Return your hands to your chest and belly, and relax.

sensory changes in the hands the most easily, so this is a good place to begin to sense qi. You may feel warmth, heaviness, or a tingling sensation. In addition you may experience pulsation, or sense a magnetic force between your fingers and palms. As you focus on the sensation in your hands, you may find that your mind becomes more peaceful and your thoughts less of a distraction. You may become more aware of your body as a whole and of the sensations, sounds, and smells of your surroundings. You may experience a heightened awareness of connection to your environment and to other people. Sensing qi is simply the state of being both relaxed and alive to the information and feeling of the moment.

SENSING QI WHILE SITTING

Sit with your body upright and relaxed, and get in touch with your breathing (*see pp18–19*). Take 3–4 minutes or more over this exercise.

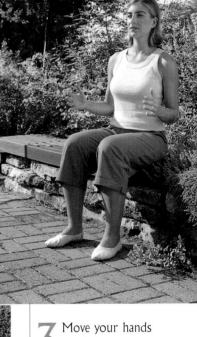

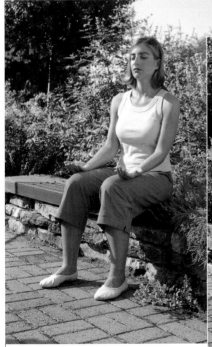

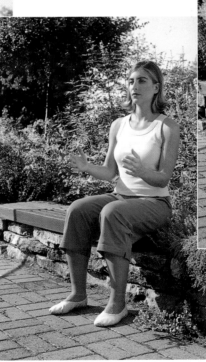

1 Place your hands on your thighs, palms up, wrists straight and relaxed. Notice any changes in sensation in your hands as you breathe in and out. Focus on the centre of both hands, then on each fingertip.

2 Keeping your elbows relaxed, raise your hands so your palms face each other, fingers pointing forwards, wrists extended and relaxed. Notice the feeling in your hands.

3 Move your hands slightly apart as you breathe in, and slightly together as you breathe out. Notice any changes in sensation as you breathe. Return your hands to your thighs, palms up, and relax.

SENSING QI WHILE STANDING

Once you can notice sensory changes in your hands in the lying and sitting positions (*see pp20–21*), move on to these standing qi exercises. They are essential for cultivating qi energy and provide the fundamental groundwork for tai chi practice. Begin and end your tai chi session with these exercises, or practise them on their own. Spend up to a minute on each position, or hold them for as long as you can comfortably stand still.

WU CHI (WUJI) POSTURE

Wu Chi, or "undivided oneness", is the standing posture most commonly practised before and after the tai chi form. It prepares you mentally and physically for tai chi by calming and focusing the mind, aligning the body, and regulating breathing and flow of qi.

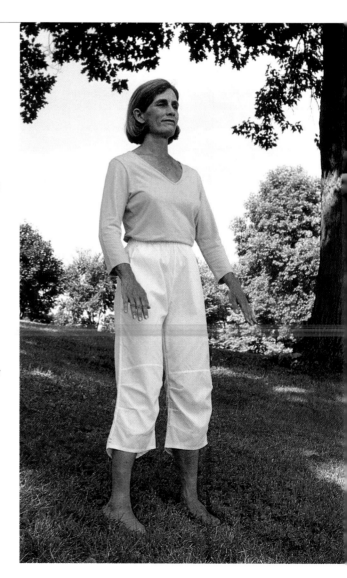

• **Stand with your feet flat,** parallel, and hip-width apart, knees slightly bent, and weight evenly distributed over both feet. Be sure to keep your lower back relaxed and spine straight.

• **Align your head** so that it feels as if it is suspended from above, and tuck your chin in very slightly. Take care not to tense your neck. Relax your jaw so that your teeth are separated and your lips just touch; the tip of your tongue lightly touches the roof of your mouth.

• **Relax your shoulders,** checking to see that they are balanced. Bend your elbows and move them slightly away from your body, creating space for a small, imaginary ball under your upper arm. Your wrists are straight and your fingers are "awake" — they point down and slightly forwards.

• **Focus** on slow, regular, and deep belly breathing (*see pp18–19*). Feel into the palms and fingers of your hands.

• **Make subtle adjustments** in your position as you begin to relax and to feel qi.

HOLDING THE BALL

Throughout the tai chi form, the hands face each other in different positions, as if holding an imaginary ball. As you practise this exercise, notice the sensation in your hands. Keep your shoulders, elbows, and wrists relaxed.

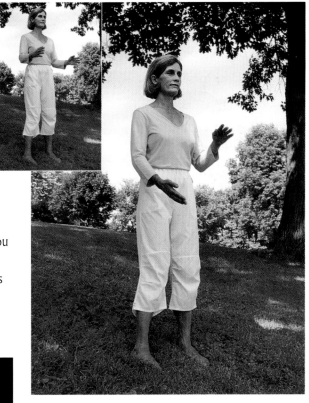

• **Stand in the Wu Chi Posture** (*see opposite*), with arms relaxed, wrists straight, and fingers awake. Bend your elbows so that your palms face each other. Notice the sensation between your hands.

• **Slowly move your hands** to the diagonal, as if you are holding an imaginary ball. Continue to move your hands around the ball, with your palms always facing each other. Maintain a sense of connection between your palms as you move your hands.

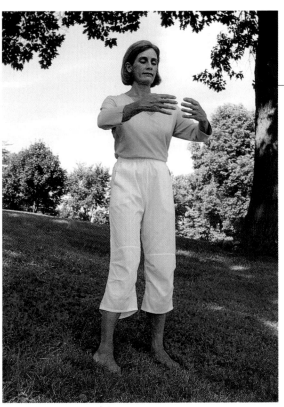

HOLDING THE MOON

You may experience a sense of connection between your fingers as you hold this position. Imagine that there is a line or an electric current between each pair of fingers and the thumbs.

• **Stand in the Wu Chi Posture** (*see opposite*), with your arms relaxed, wrists extended, and fingers awake.

• **Position your arms** in front of your body as if they are encircling a large imaginary ball. Your fingertips face each other, without touching, at midline.

• **Your thumbs** point to each other, forming the shape of a crescent moon between fingers and thumbs.

• **Make sure** that each finger and thumb faces its mate on the other hand.

• **Be sure** to keep your neck, shoulders, and elbows relaxed and heavy.

WARMING UP

These exercises prepare your body and mind for tai chi practice. They will help you develop flexibility and strength in your back, chest, pelvis, shoulders, and hips, and promote the flow of qi in these areas. Move gently and slowly, paying attention to your own physical cues. Practise all of these exercises in sequence, focusing more time on areas that you feel need more attention.

THE WATERFALL

This exercise helps to lengthen and strengthen the muscles of your neck and back, which are structurally two of the most vulnerable areas of the body. Practise the movement slowly in a smooth, continuous flow.

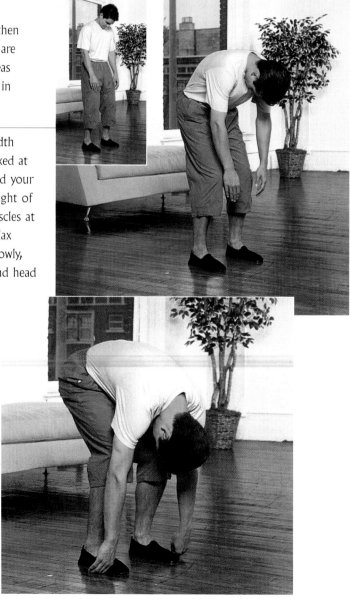

1 Stand with your feet parallel and hip-width apart, knees slightly bent, and arms relaxed at your sides. Let your head hang forwards and your arms dangle relaxed and heavy. Feel the weight of your head and arms gently stretch the muscles at the back of your neck and upper back. Relax your jaw, and breathe. Then curl forward slowly, keeping your knees bent and your arms and head relaxed. Allow the weight of your head, arms, and shoulders to loosen the muscles of your back as you descend.

2 Curl down as far as is comfortable, then slowly uncurl, focusing on each vertebra in your spine and keeping your knees bent and head and arms heavy. Slowly return to the upright starting position. Repeat the entire movement at least 5 times.

THE FROG STANCE

This resting position is otherwise known as squatting. It helps lengthen the muscles of the lower back, which relieves stress on the lumbar vertebrae. Moving into and out of the squat strengthens the quadriceps, the large muscles at the fronts of the thighs. It also increases ankle flexibility and lengthens the calf muscles, both of which are important for maintaining balance. Once you are comfortable in the standard Frog Stance, progress to the weight-shifting exercise.

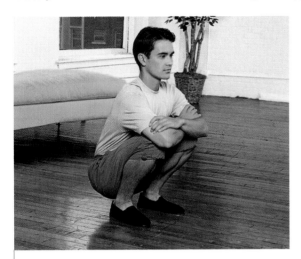

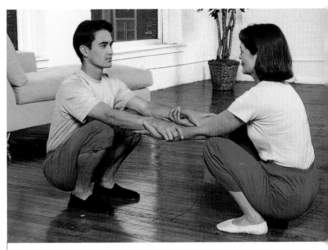

Stand with your feet parallel or in an open "V" position. Bend your knees and slowly lower yourself down into the squatting position. Keep both heels flat on the floor to prevent strain on the knees. If you can't do a full squat, bend down as far as you feel comfortable. Hold the squat for as long as you can, then stand up. Repeat 1–2 times.

You can practise squatting using a partner for support; however, choose a person who is similar to you in height and weight. Each person holds the partner's wrist — one from the top, the other from below. You can also hold a door frame or doorknob for stability.

Shifting weight in the frog stance. This improves ankle flexibility, stretches the calves and lower back, and strengthens the quadriceps. Once you are comfortable squatting with your feet flat, begin shifting a little of your weight back and forth from one foot to the other. Keeping your heels on the floor, shift all of your weight on to one foot and balance there for 2–3 seconds, or as long as is comfortable. Repeat 3–4 times, then stand up.

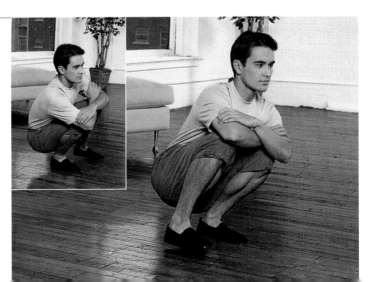

THE BELLY ROLL

This exercise helps to isolate the movement of the pelvis and increase flexibility in the lower back, which can help to improve posture. As you become aware of the mobility in your pelvis, you can begin to make subtle adjustments in that area that relieve strain on your back and transfer weight to your legs instead. To begin with, it may help to practise these exercises in front of a mirror.

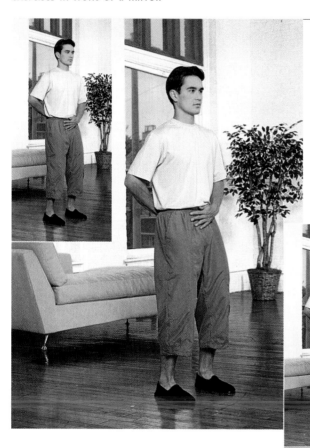

1 Stand with your feet hip-width apart and knees slightly bent. Place one hand on your belly and the other on your back. Then, tilt your pelvis forwards and back without moving your head, shoulders, or knees. Be sure not to straighten your knees. Repeat this slowly 3–5 times.

2 Once you are comfortable moving your pelvis forwards and back, try moving it from side to side. Repeat this about 3–5 times, then try moving your pelvis in a circular motion, first 2–3 times in one direction, and then 2–3 times in the other.

CRANE SPREADS WINGS

This exercise is based on an ancient qigong exercise for energizing the heart and lungs. It helps open up the back and chest. It also stimulates the middle *dan tian*, the energy field located in the chest (*see pp146–147*). First practise holding the positions as described, then try moving in a slow, continuous flow.

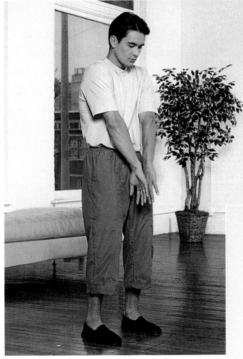

1 Stand with your feet hip-width apart, knees slightly bent, and arms relaxed at your sides. Round your shoulders forwards, bringing the backs of your hands together, if possible. Pause and relax into this position. Breathe in, feeling the increased stretch in your upper back. Hold this position for one full breath in and out.

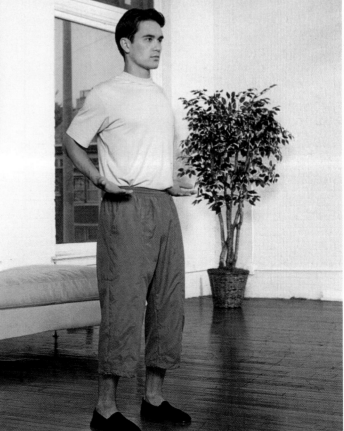

2 Roll your shoulders back, bending your elbows so that your palms face up. Pause and relax into this position. Breathe in, feeling the increased stretch in your chest. Hold this position for one full breath in and out. Repeat the entire movement 2–3 times.

SOAR ABOVE THE CLOUDS

Everyday activities, such as cooking, cleaning, sitting at a computer, or even swinging a hammer, can cause the shoulders to round forwards. This depresses the chest and inhibits natural breathing. Practise this exercise to help open the shoulders and chest and align the head with the body.

1 Stand with your feet hip-width apart and knees slightly bent. Raise your arms to shoulder height at your sides, with hands facing forwards and elbows slightly bent. Tuck in your chin very slightly, relax, and hold the position for 2–5 seconds. Then slowly move your arms back, and feel the stretch in your shoulders, arms, and chest. Take a deep breath, and relax into this position, holding it for 2–5 seconds.

2 Bring your arms slightly forwards, still at shoulder height with hands facing forwards, and hold for 2–5 seconds. Repeat the entire movement 3–4 times.

STAND FIRM AND EMBRACE THE SKY

This movement promotes hip flexibility and leg strength while expanding the shoulders and rib cage upwards. As you practise this, maintain the feeling of standing firm and stable as you extend your energy out into your hands and above.

1 Stand with feet in an open "V" position, knees slightly bent and aligned over your toes. Check that your lower back is straight. Allow your arms to hang at your sides, fingers extended and pointing out and down. Hold this position for a few seconds to one minute initially, then for longer.

2 Keeping your legs bent, raise your arms above your head so that your fingers point out and up. Feel the stretch in your torso and ribs. Keep your shoulders relaxed, and your back straight. Hold this position for a few seconds or up to a few minutes.

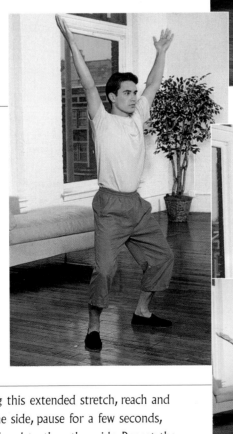

3 Maintaining this extended stretch, reach and bend to one side, pause for a few seconds, then reach and bend to the other side. Repeat the movement 2–3 times on each side. Finally, return to the centre, slowly lower your hands, straighten your knees, and take a few relaxed breaths.

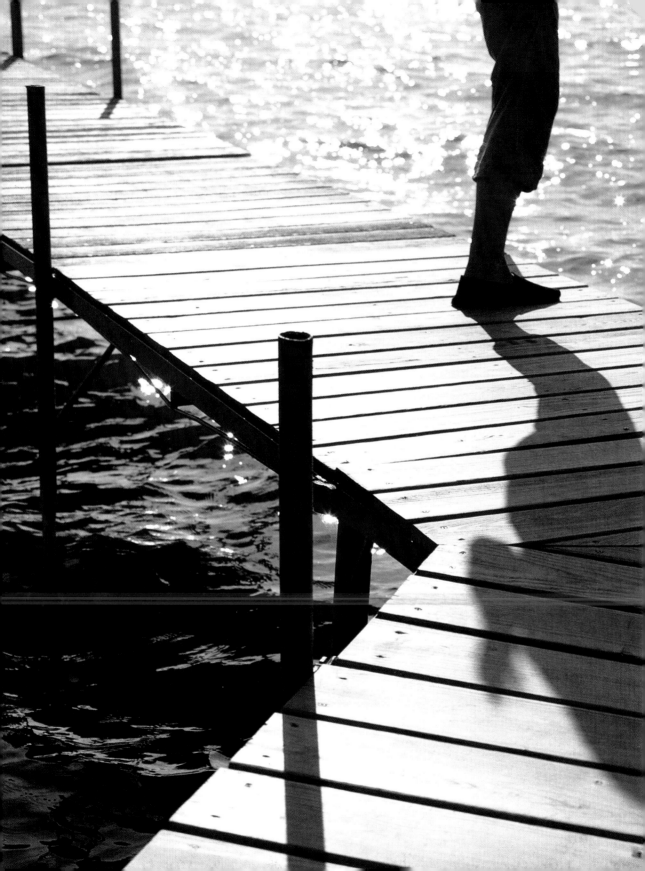

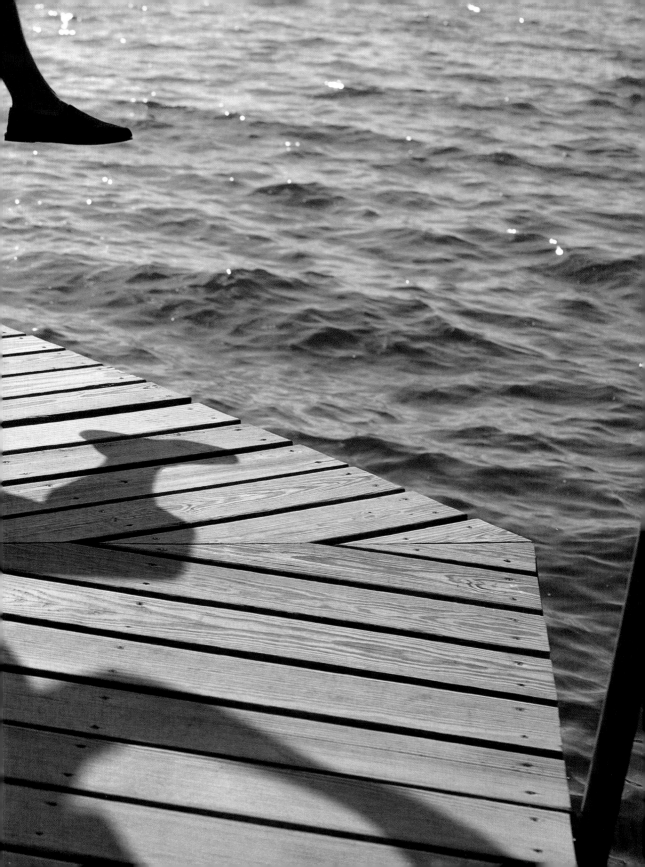

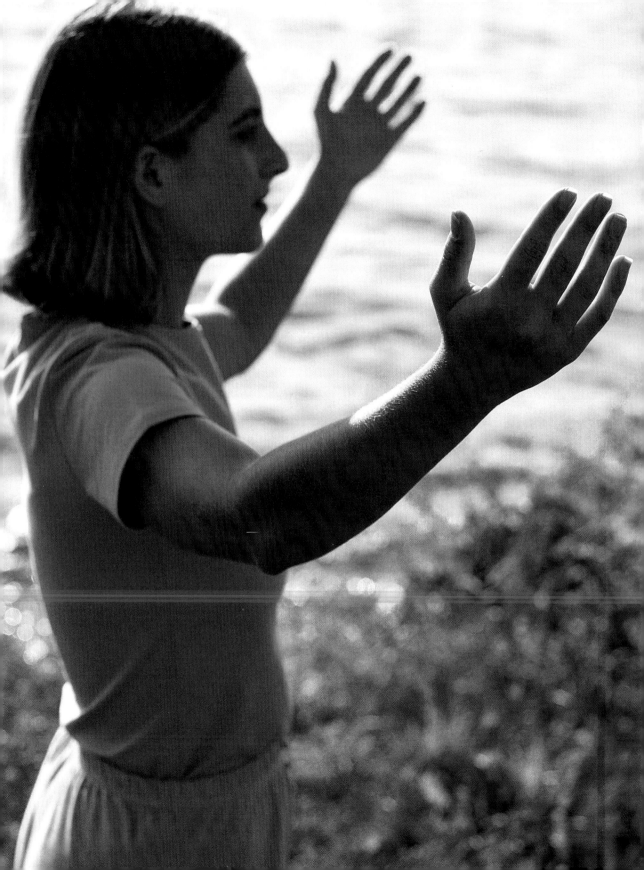

BASIC MOVES

These exercises train you to move correctly when practising tai chi.
They also provide practice in coordinating breathing with movement and
staying relaxed and aware of qi while in motion. Each movement integrates
the skills from the preceding movement and progresses in difficulty.
Basic Moves is divided into three parts. Learn the movements in an
entire part before attempting the corresponding part in the Form.
Ideally, you should practise sensing qi and breathing (*see pp18–23*),
and warm up (*see pp24–29*) before you begin.

PART ONE

Here you learn the movements that you will encounter in Part One of the Form.
They provide the foundation for moving comfortably and effectively within your
body's natural range of motion. Practise these exercises in a flowing sequence, or stop
and hold positions. Move slowly and gently; embrace the moment.

HORSE STANCE

This position is the foundation for tai chi movement. Stand in a relaxed manner with your body upright and naturally aligned as you focus on breathing slowly and deeply. This promotes the relaxed, alert state of mind and body essential for tai chi practice.

BENEFITS Strengthens deeper structural or "core" muscles that help natural alignment; keeping knees slightly bent engages thigh muscles and stabilizes knees.

TIP Be aware of the soles of your feet – this is essential for feeling "grounded" or connected with the earth.

gaze forwards with awareness of the periphery

keep shoulders relaxed and straight

lengthen and open the back of your neck

slightly lower your chin

weight is evenly distributed over both feet

knees are slightly bent

FRONT VIEW

Stand with feet flat, parallel, and hip-width apart and your arms relaxed at your sides. Your knees are soft, slightly bent, and your weight is evenly distributed over both feet. Your mouth is closed with your lips slightly touching; the tip of your tongue touches the roof of your mouth. Relax your belly as you breathe slowly, gently, and deeply through your nose. Stand like this for 1 minute or more.

SIDE VIEW

With your knees slightly bent, allow your pelvis to relax and hang in a neutral position. Your tailbone is aligned with your heels, and your head feels as if it is suspended from above.

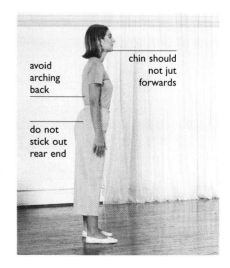

avoid arching back

chin should not jut forwards

do not stick out rear end

POINTS TO WATCH

• **Stand straight**, your tailbone aligned with your heels; otherwise, you put unnecessary strain on your lower back.

• **Keep your belly relaxed** to help you to breathe deeply.
• **Relax your chin and jaw** to aid your natural alignment.

HEAVY ARMS

Although our arms hang from our shoulders, we often tend to unconsciously tense them. This exercise helps you to relax your arms and to become aware of their weight. Based in qigong, it is the starting point for learning to use minimal effort in all tai chi arm movement and for sensing qi.

BENEFITS Releases tension in the neck and shoulders; replenishes fluid in the shoulder joints.

TIP Imagine that your arms are heavy like ropes or pendulums.

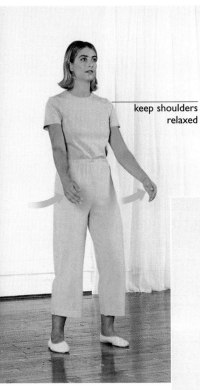

keep shoulders relaxed

1 Stand in the *Horse Stance* with feet hip-width apart and arms relaxed by your sides. Swing your arms forwards, taking care not to tense your neck and shoulders.

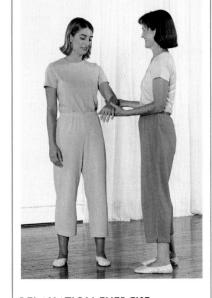

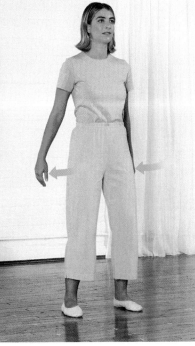

2 Then swing your arms back. As your shoulders and elbows become more relaxed, swing higher. Repeat 10 times, then return to the *Horse Stance* with arms by your sides.

RELAXATION EXERCISE
Practise this exercise with a partner. Completely relax your arm at your side. Allow your partner to lift your arm, supporting it at the elbow and wrist. When you are relaxed, your arm will feel extremely heavy to your partner. When you tense your arm, it will feel much lighter. Practise keeping your arm completely relaxed as your partner lifts and gently moves it around.

RIDING THE HORSE

In tai chi, all movements in the legs involve relaxing into the hips, knees, and ankles. This exercise trains you to keep your body upright and relaxed as you bend your knees. Placing your hands on your belly and back helps you to feel the position of your pelvis and torso.

BENEFITS Strengthens thigh muscles, which minimizes stress to the knees; increases ankle flexibility; improves balance.

TIPS Movement is rooted in the feet and powered by the legs; to help your posture, imagine that you are balancing a book on your head.

1 Stand in the *Horse Stance* with feet hip-width apart and knees soft. Keep your feet flat and your weight evenly distributed over both feet. Place one hand on your belly and the other on your lower back. Take a few moments to breathe slowly and naturally. Remember to keep your lower back relaxed and feel as though your head is suspended from above.

At a glance

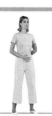 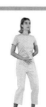 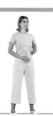 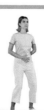 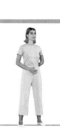

Weight centre.......Bend..........Straighten.........Bend......Straighten..Repeat

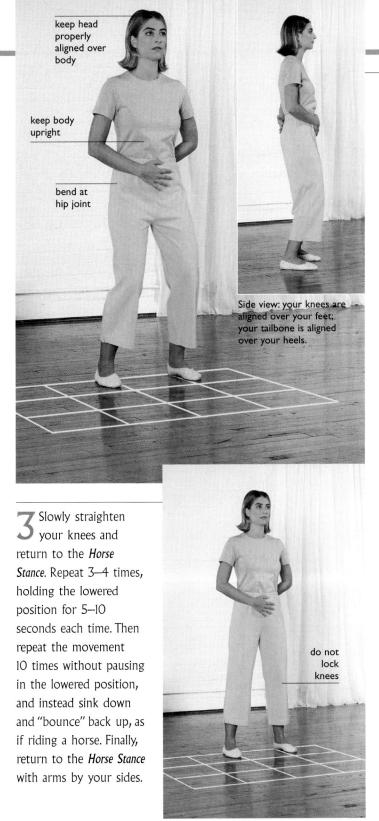

keep head properly aligned over body

keep body upright

bend at hip joint

Side view: your knees are aligned over your feet; your tailbone is aligned over your heels.

2 Keeping your body upright and your back straight, slowly bend your knees and lower your body down. Hold this position for 5–10 seconds, feeling into your feet. Make sure that your weight is evenly distributed over the soles of both feet, not concentrated on the balls of your feet or your toes.

POINTS TO WATCH

• **Do not** allow your knees to extend beyond your toes.
• **Avoid** rounding or arching the back, or collapsing the chest, since this will affect your balance.
• **Keep** your back straight, since this minimizes stress to the back.

3 Slowly straighten your knees and return to the *Horse Stance*. Repeat 3–4 times, holding the lowered position for 5–10 seconds each time. Then repeat the movement 10 times without pausing in the lowered position, and instead sink down and "bounce" back up, as if riding a horse. Finally, return to the *Horse Stance* with arms by your sides.

do not lock knees

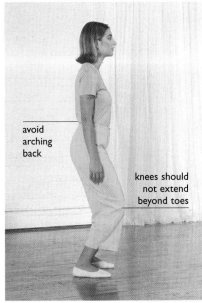

avoid arching back

knees should not extend beyond toes

CRANE TAKES FLIGHT

This exercise combines *Riding the Horse* with *Heavy Arms* in a relaxed, flowing manner that is characteristic of all tai chi movement. Based on ancient qigong exercises for the heart and lungs, it is inspired by the graceful movement of the crane flapping its wings in flight. Let the arm movements follow your natural breathing.

BENEFITS Coordinating movement with breathing enhances the flow of qi in the body; arm movements add a cardiovascular benefit.

TIPS Feel light, unrestrained, uplifted; inhale as you raise your arms, exhale as you lower them.

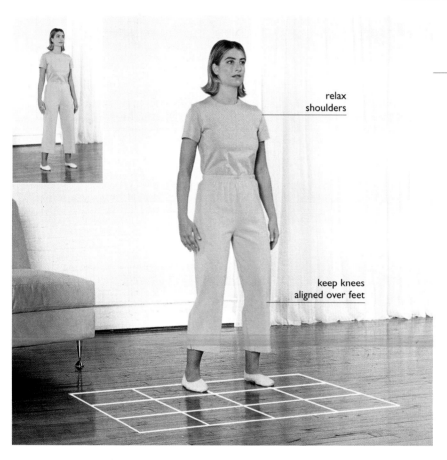

relax shoulders

keep knees aligned over feet

1 Stand in the *Horse Stance* with feet hip-width apart, knees soft, and arms relaxed at your sides. Then slowly bend your knees, keeping your tailbone in alignment with your heels, as you raise your arms very slightly. Breathe slowly and deeply.

At a glance

    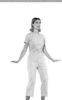

Breathe naturally...Exhale...Inhale to raise arms...Exhale to lower arms...Repeat

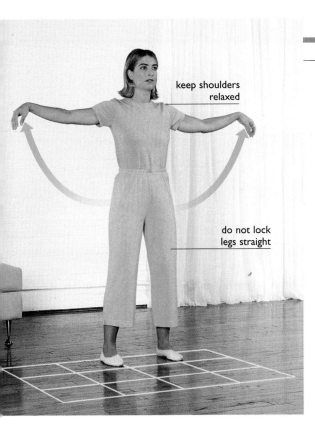

keep shoulders
relaxed

do not lock
legs straight

2 Slowly straighten your knees and return to the *Horse Stance* as you inhale and raise your hands to shoulder height at your sides. Allow your wrists to lead the movement, but keep your hands relaxed.

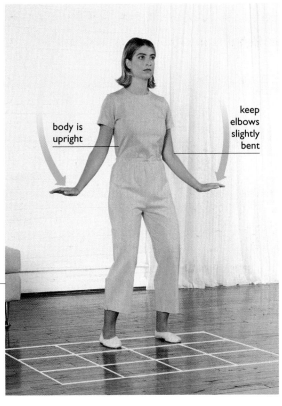

body is
upright

keep
elbows
slightly
bent

3 Exhale as you bend your knees and slowly lower your arms, leading with your wrists. Keep your neck and shoulders relaxed. Repeat the movement 10 times, then return to the *Horse Stance* with arms by your sides.

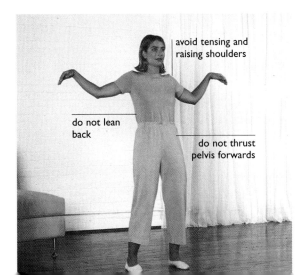

avoid tensing and
raising shoulders

do not lean
back

do not thrust
pelvis forwards

POINTS TO WATCH

- **Keep** your shoulders relaxed; otherwise, you create tension in the neck.
- **Stand straight** with your body upright in order to minimize stress to the back.

- **Relax** your lower back so that your pelvis hangs in a neutral position and your back is straight.
- **Raise** your arms to the same height at your sides for balance

BEAR ROOTS ON ONE LEG

This movement introduces weight separation: establishing a stable base of support or "root" on one foot while keeping your body relaxed, balanced, and aligned. To begin with, practise keeping both feet on the floor as you shift your weight until you feel stable on one foot.

BENEFITS Strengthens thigh and hip muscles; improves balance; strengthens and stabilizes spine; trains you to keep shoulders relaxed when stressed; promotes correct positioning of hands and wrists for tai chi movement.

TIP Imagine that your hands are resting on two poles for balance.

1 Stand in the *Horse Stance* with feet hip-width apart and knees soft. Bend your elbows so that your forearms are parallel to the floor.

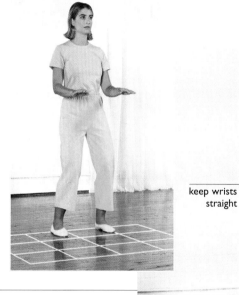

keep shoulders relaxed and balanced

keep wrists straight

keep hips even

weight is evenly distributed over entire sole of foot

2 Slowly shift your weight entirely on to your left foot, keeping your left knee aligned over your left foot. Then lift your right foot just barely off the floor for 1–10 seconds. Keep your shoulders relaxed and balanced, your forearms parallel to the floor, and your arms and hands relaxed.

At a glance

    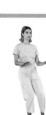

Weight centre...Shift left.....Shift right....Shift left......Shift right..Repeat

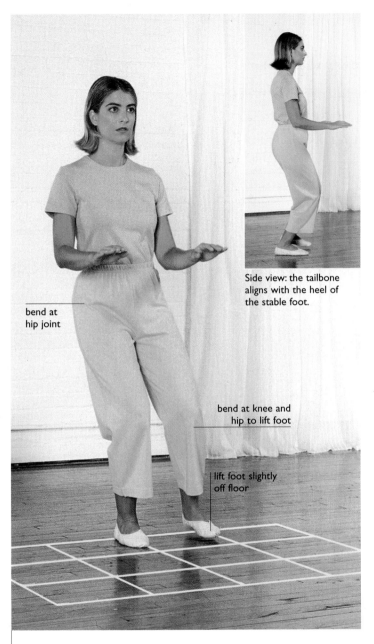

bend at
hip joint

Side view: the tailbone
aligns with the heel of
the stable foot.

bend at knee and
hip to lift foot

lift foot slightly
off floor

POINTS TO WATCH

- **Keep** the knee of your stable leg aligned over your toes.
- **Avoid** sticking out your hip, since this puts unnecessary strain on your hips.
- **Do not tilt** your body to one side – this puts strain on your lower back.
- **Do not lift** your foot too high off the floor; lift your foot just high enough to take your weight off it.

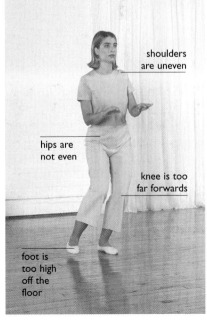

shoulders
are uneven

hips are
not even

knee is too
far forwards

foot is
too high
off the
floor

3 Slowly shift your weight entirely on to your right foot, and lift your left foot off the floor. Take care to keep your hips straight and your body upright at all times. Repeat the movement 5 times on each side, slowly taking time to balance for 1–10 seconds, then return to the *Horse Stance* with arms by your sides.

STABLE AND OPEN

This movement trains you to keep your knee properly aligned over your weight-bearing foot when making transitions in tai chi. One leg supports your weight as you turn your torso and pelvis outwards in the direction of your unweighted foot. Remember to keep your back straight and your body upright.

BENEFITS Improves balance; increases flexibility of groin muscles; strengthens hip and thigh muscles.

TIP During the turning movement, sense a connection between your tailbone and the heel of your weight-bearing foot.

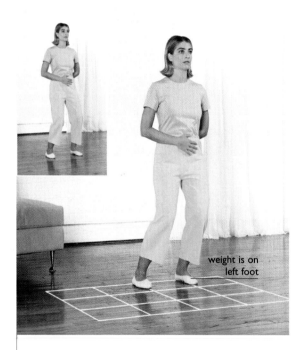

weight is on left foot

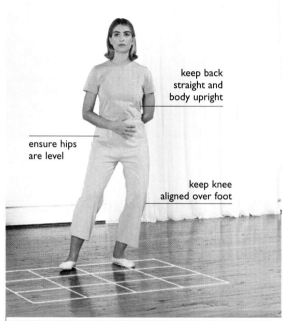

keep back straight and body upright

ensure hips are level

keep knee aligned over foot

1 Stand in the *Horse Stance* with feet hip-width apart and knees soft. Place one hand on your belly and the other on your lower back. Then shift your weight entirely on to your left foot.

2 Keeping your weight entirely on your left foot, move into *Stable and Open* by turning your pelvis, torso, right leg, and foot outwards at a 45° angle, pivoting on your heel. Keep your head aligned with your pelvis.

At a glance

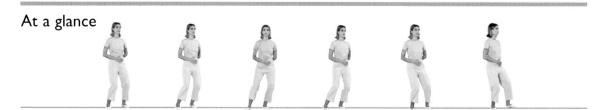

Weight centre..Shift left..Turn right..Turn centre..Shift right..Turn left..Repeat

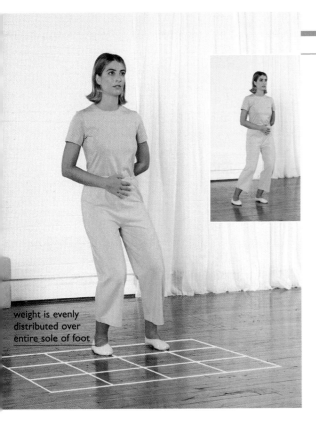

weight is evenly
distributed over
entire sole of foot

3 Keep all your weight on your left foot as you turn your pelvis, torso, right leg, and foot inwards so that your right foot is parallel to your left foot and flat on the ground. Then shift your weight entirely on to your right foot.

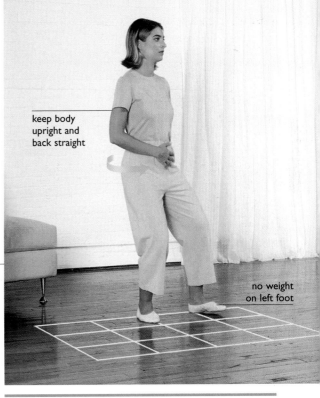

keep body
upright and
back straight

no weight
on left foot

4 Keeping all your weight on your right foot, move into *Stable and Open* by turning your pelvis, torso, left leg, and foot outwards at a 45° angle, pivoting on your heel. Repeat 5 times, then return to the *Horse Stance* with arms by your sides.

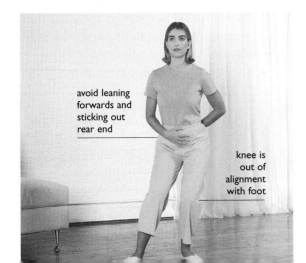

avoid leaning
forwards and
sticking out
rear end

knee is
out of
alignment
with foot

POINTS TO WATCH

• **Keep** your body upright and your back straight. If you tend to lean forwards, you probably have tight groin muscles – practise *Gathering the Stars* (pp44–45) in addition to this exercise to help stretch these muscles.

• **Keep** the knee of your weight-bearing leg aligned over your foot. Do not allow your knee to extend beyond your toe.

• **Avoid** tilting your hips.

GATHERING THE STARS

Here, the pivoting action from *Stable and Open* is combined with expressive arm movements. Practise coordinating your breathing with your arm movements: breathe in as you open your arms, and breathe out as you gather your arms towards you.

> **BENEFITS** Aligns neck vertebrae; builds arm strength; expands muscles in chest; opening the arms can have an uplifting effect; provides practice in sensing qi while moving.
>
> **TIP** As you open your arms, imagine that you are reaching out to embrace the stars.

fingers face but do not touch

1 Stand in the *Horse Stance* with feet hip-width apart, knees soft, and arms in front of you in the *Holding the Moon* position (*see p23*). Focus on breathing slowly and deeply.

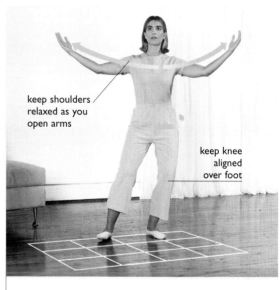

keep shoulders relaxed as you open arms

keep knee aligned over foot

2 Shift your weight entirely on to your left foot as you slowly exhale.

3 Keeping all your weight on your left leg, move into *Stable and Open* by turning your pelvis, torso, right leg, and foot outwards at a 45° angle, pivoting on your heel. As you do this, breathe in slowly and open your arms.

At a glance

Breathe naturally...Exhale...Inhale to open arms...Exhale to close arms......Repeat

4 Keeping all your weight on your left foot, turn your pelvis, torso, and right leg forwards so that your right foot is parallel to your left foot and flat on the ground. Simultaneously begin breathing out, and bring your arms back into the *Holding the Moon* position.

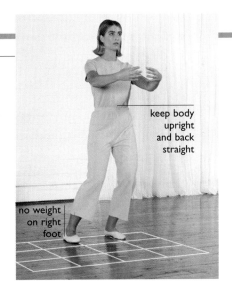

keep body upright and back straight

no weight on right foot

5 Shift your weight entirely on to your right foot, keeping your arms in the *Holding the Moon* position, as you continue to exhale.

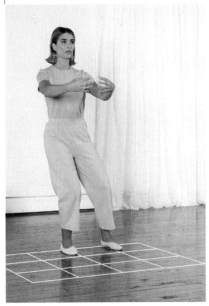

keep shoulders and hips aligned

keep knee aligned over foot

no weight on left foot

6 Move into *Stable and Open* by turning your pelvis, torso, left leg, and foot outwards at a 45° angle, pivoting on your heel. Simultaneously inhale slowly as you open your arms. Repeat the movement 5 times on each side, then return to the *Horse Stance* with arms by your sides.

THE TAI CHI STANCE

Characteristic of Yang-Style tai chi, this essential stance provides a wide base of support that maximizes stability when shifting weight. It is also known as the 70/30 Stance because when the weight is forward, 70 percent is on the front foot and 30 percent is on the back foot. When the weight is on the back foot, it supports the entire weight of the body.

BENEFITS Strengthens thighs; improves balance; increases ankle flexibility; lengthens calf muscles.

TIP Practise balancing in this stance when standing on a moving bus, subway, or boat.

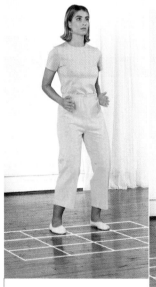

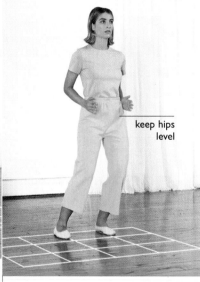

keep hips level

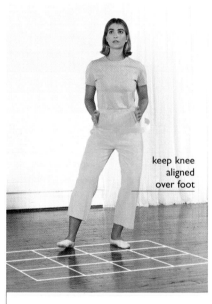

keep knee aligned over foot

1 Stand in the *Horse Stance* with feet hip-width apart and knees soft. Place your hands at your hips, fingers pointing forwards.

2 Slowly shift your weight on to your left leg, taking care to keep your knee aligned over your foot.

3 Move into *Stable and Open* by turning your pelvis, torso, right leg, and foot outwards at a 45° angle, pivoting on your heel. Take care not to arch your back.

At a glance

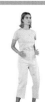   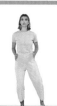

Weight centre.........Shift left..............Turn right................Shift right.....

4 Shift all of your weight on to your right, diagonal foot.

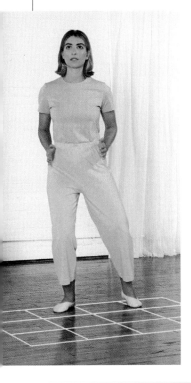

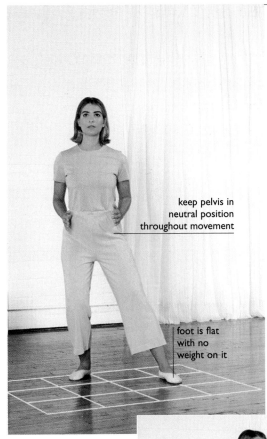

keep pelvis in neutral position throughout movement

foot is flat with no weight on it

5 Keeping all of your weight on your right foot, step directly forwards, heel first, with your left foot into the *Tai Chi Stance, Back Position.* Your feet should be hip-width apart.

6 Shift 70 percent of your weight forwards on to your front, left foot, keeping your knee aligned over your foot. Simultaneously turn your torso and pelvis to face forwards. This is the *Tai Chi Stance, Forward Position.* Repeat 3–4 times, or until you feel comfortable with the move. Then step back, return to the start position, and repeat on the other side. Finally return to the *Horse Stance* with arms by your sides.

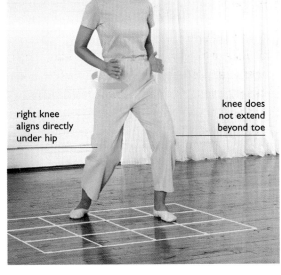

right knee aligns directly under hip

knee does not extend beyond toe

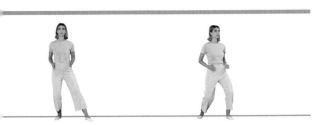

...Step forwards...........Shift/Turn...Repeat

BEAR MOVES WITH CRANE ARMS

This movement provides practice in shifting weight forwards and back in the *Tai Chi Stance*. Keep your body upright and your feet flat during the weight shift, and aim to keep your body at the same height throughout the movement. Practise synchronizing your breathing with your arm movements.

BENEFITS Arm movements add a cardiovascular benefit and strengthen the upper body; synchronizing breathing with movement has an energizing effect.

TIP Keep arms relaxed to help feel qi in the fingertips as you move.

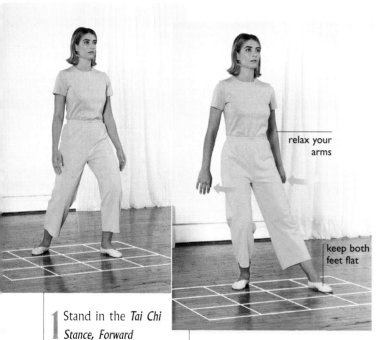

relax your arms

keep both feet flat

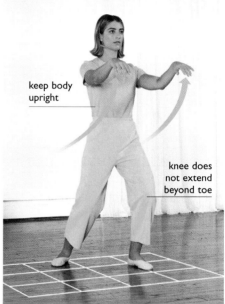

keep body upright

knee does not extend beyond toe

1 Stand in the *Tai Chi Stance, Forward Position*, with 70 percent of your weight on your right, front foot and your arms by your sides. Breathe.

2 Move into the *Tai Chi Stance, Back Position* by shifting all of your weight on to your back foot. Exhale slowly as you swing your arms back.

3 Move into the *Tai Chi Stance, Forward Position*, by shifting 70 percent of your weight on to your front foot. As you do this, inhale slowly and swing your arms to shoulder height in front of you.

At a glance

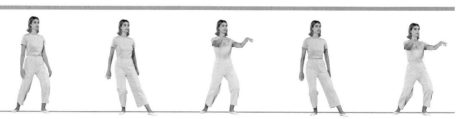

Breathe naturally........Inhale to raise arms....Exhale to lower arms.....Repeat

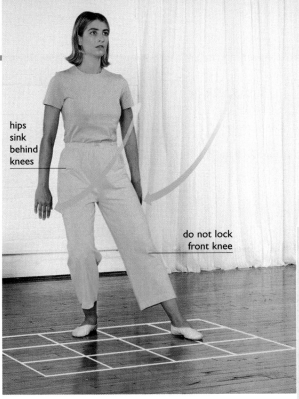

hips
sink
behind
knees

do not lock
front knee

4 Exhale slowly, and move into the *Tai Chi Stance, Back Position,* by shifting all of your weight on to your back foot as you swing your arms back. Maintain the same height as you shift back.

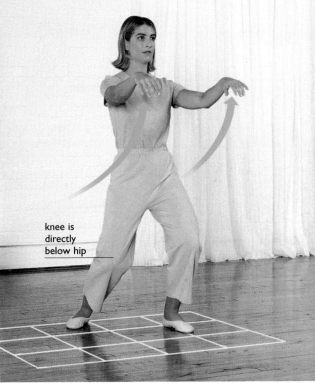

knee is
directly
below hip

5 Move into the *Tai Chi Stance, Forward Position* by shifting 70 percent of your weight on to your front foot as you inhale slowly and raise your arms to shoulder height in front of you. Repeat 4–5 times, then practise with the right foot forward. Finally, move feet parallel and relax.

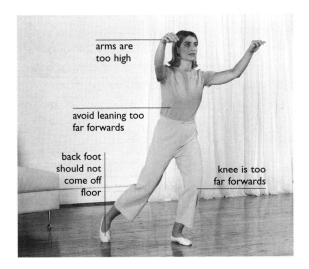

arms are
too high

avoid leaning too
far forwards

back foot
should not
come off
floor

knee is too
far forwards

POINTS TO WATCH

- **Do not lean** too far forwards when weight is forward, since this will affect balance.
- **Keep** your front knee aligned over the toe of your stable foot; otherwise, you risk straining your knee.
- **The back foot** does not come off the floor.
- **Do not swing** your arms higher than shoulder height in front of you. Keep your shoulders relaxed.

TAI CHI STANCE FORWARD TRANSITION

This movement provides practice in transitioning forwards while maintaining the wide, stable base of the *Tai Chi Stance*. Step as far forwards as you can, keeping your body upright and all of your weight on your back foot.

> **BENEFITS** Good practice in maintaining body alignment and balance in a wide stance.
>
> **TIP** Combine this with the shifting motion and arms from *Bear Moves with Crane Arms* (pp48–49).

foot is at a 45° angle.

hips face forward

fingers indicate direction pelvis faces

hips still face forwards

keep knee bent

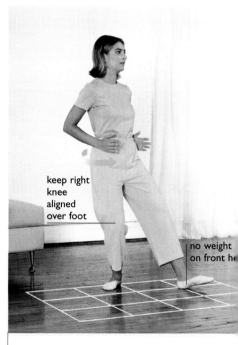

keep right knee aligned over foot

no weight on front he[...]

1 Stand in the *Tai Chi Stance, Forward Position*, with 70 percent of your weight on your left, front foot and your hands at your hips, fingers pointing forwards. Your right, back foot is positioned diagonally outward at a 45° angle.

2 Move into the *Tai Chi Stance, Back Position*, by shifting all of your weight on to your right, back foot.

3 Keeping your weight entirely on your right foot, rotate your pelvis, torso, left leg, and foot outwards at a 45° angle, pivoting on your heel.

At a glance

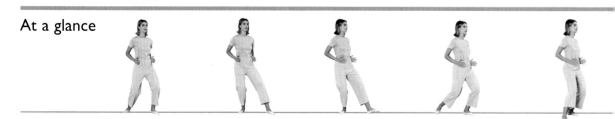

Weight forwards....Shift back........Turn left.....Shift forwards...Step forward

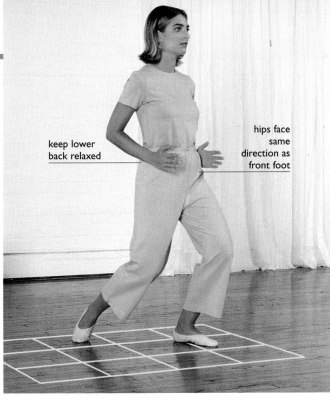

keep lower
back relaxed

hips face
same
direction as
front foot

4 Shift all of your weight forwards on to your left, front foot to move into the *Forward Transition*.

5 Keeping your weight entirely on your left foot, step forwards with your right foot into the *Tai Chi Stance*. Your torso still faces the same direction as your left, back foot.

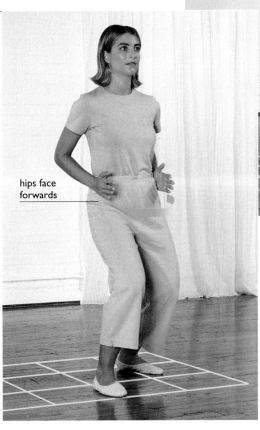

hips face
forwards

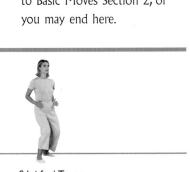

6 Move into the *Tai Chi Stance, Forward Position*, by aligning your right knee over your foot, then shifting 70 percent of your weight on to your right, front foot as you turn your pelvis and torso to face forwards. Continue moving forwards by repeating steps 2–6 on the other side. Repeat 3–4 times or until comfortable with the sequence, then move feet parallel and relax. Continue to Basic Moves Section 2, or you may end here.

hips still
face
direction
of left
foot

no weight
on front
foot

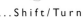

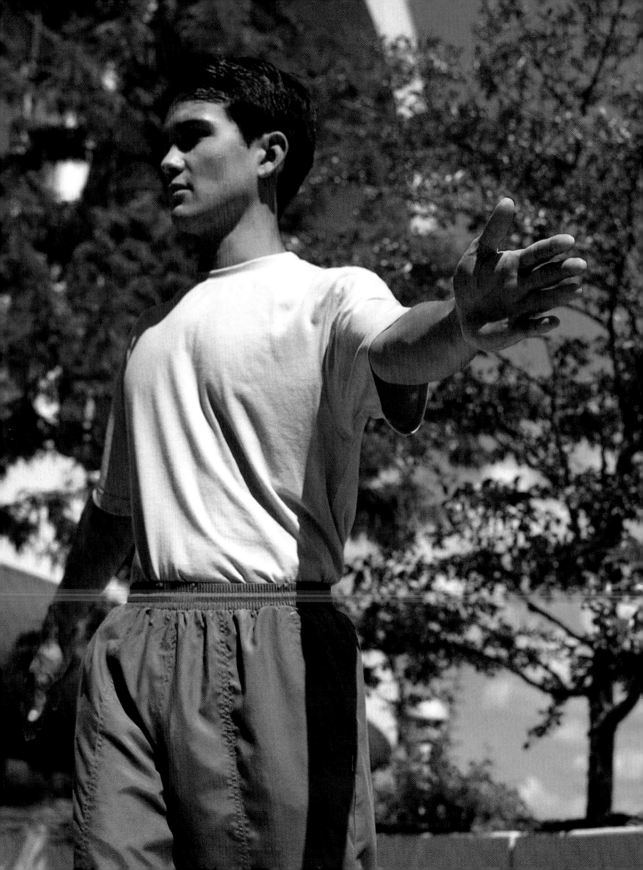

BASIC MOVES

PART TWO

This part builds on skills learned in Part One and introduces movements found in Part Two of the Form. Here you learn the *Tai Chi Fold*, a powerful wind-up motion that involves turning your pelvis and torso. This part also provides practice in some of tai chi's more complex footwork. Learn the moves in this part before attempting Part Two of the Form. Keep your body aligned, centred, and stable, and your movements circular, smooth, and loose.

THE TAI CHI FOLD

This is a powerful wind-up motion that occurs naturally when throwing or pushing, for example, or when playing sports such as tennis or golf. It is a fundamental tai chi move that essentially involves rotating your pelvis and torso. Here you learn to execute the move correctly by breaking down the basic mechanics. In loose clothing, this movement causes a diagonal "fold" at the hip joint or *kwa*.

> **BENEFITS** Increases hip flexibility; trains correct movement when pushing, pulling, hitting, throwing, and blocking.
>
> **TIP** Your knees must be slightly bent in order to perform the move correctly.

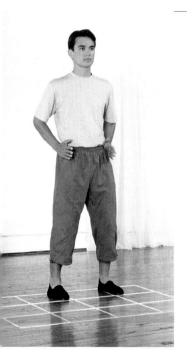

1 Stand in the *Horse Stance* with feet hip-width apart, knees slightly bent, and hands at your hips with fingers pointing forwards.

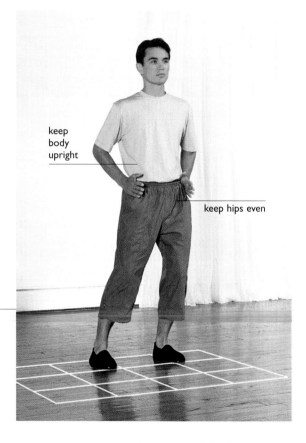

keep body upright

keep hips even

2 Slowly shift your weight entirely on to your left foot. Keep your weight evenly distributed over the sole of your foot.

At a glance

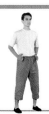 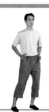 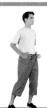 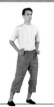 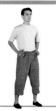 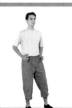

Weight centre...Shift left...Turn left...Turn centre...Shift centre...Shift right

3 With your weight entirely on your left foot, turn your pelvis and torso to the left, keeping both of your feet flat on the floor. This movement is the *Tai Chi Fold*.

4 Keeping your weight on your left foot and your body upright, turn your pelvis and torso to face forwards.

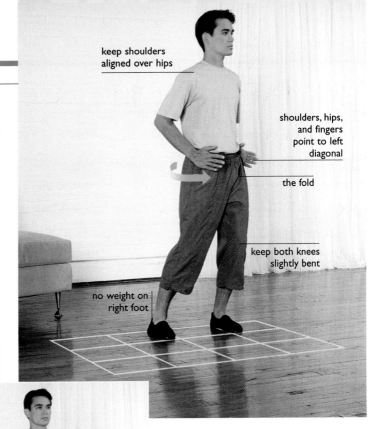

keep shoulders aligned over hips

shoulders, hips, and fingers point to left diagonal

the fold

keep both knees slightly bent

no weight on right foot

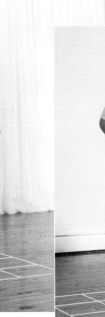

weight on right foot

POINTS TO WATCH

- **Keep** your body upright; don't lean forwards – this affects your alignment.
- **Both feet** remain flat on the floor throughout the movement.
- **Keep** your hips straight.
- **Move** your torso and pelvis as a unit; don't twist your torso.

5 Shift your weight back to the centre so that it is evenly distributed over both feet in the *Horse Stance*. Repeat the sequence of movements 4–5 times on each side, then return to the *Horse Stance* with arms by your sides.

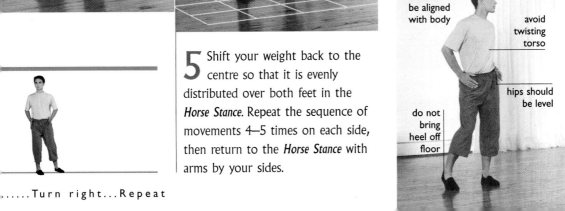

head should be aligned with body

avoid twisting torso

hips should be level

do not bring heel off floor

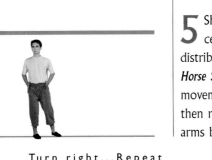

......Turn right...Repeat

MOVING THE MOON

Adding the *Holding the Moon* arm position to the basic *Tai Chi Fold*, this exercise provides practice in keeping your shoulders aligned over your hips as you execute the fold. Take care not to move your arms or shoulders independently of your hips and torso. Keep your fingers aligned with the centre of your chest.

BENEFITS Can help prevent back injuries when turning; builds strength and endurance in shoulders and arms.

TIPS Practise this as a moving qigong exercise; keep your fingers aligned in the *Holding the Moon* position to maintain the flow of qi.

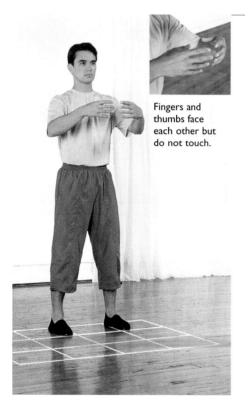

Fingers and thumbs face each other but do not touch.

1 Stand in the *Horse Stance* with feet hip-width apart and knees soft. Raise your arms in front of you as if holding a large ball, with fingers and thumbs facing each other, in the *Holding the Moon* position (*see p23*).

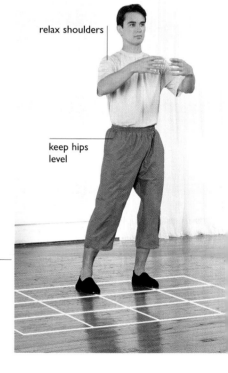

relax shoulders

keep hips level

2 Shift your weight entirely on to your left foot, keeping your hips level and your lower back relaxed.

At a glance

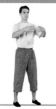 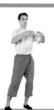 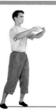 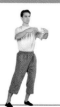 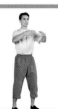

Weight centre.....Shift left......Turn left.....Turn centre...Shift centre.....

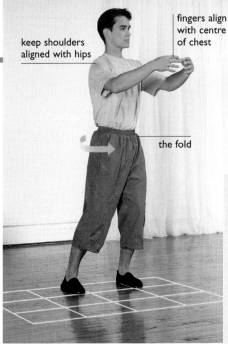

keep shoulders
aligned with hips

fingers align
with centre
of chest

the fold

3 Fold to the left by turning your pelvis and torso to the left as you sink your weight entirely on to your left leg. Keep your arms in the same position in front of the body.

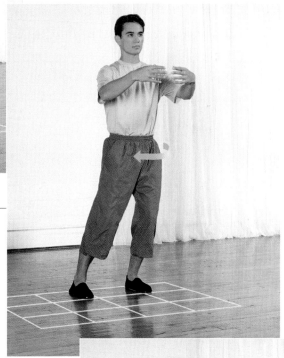

4 With your weight still on your left leg, turn your pelvis and torso to the centre, maintaining the arm position. Keep your shoulders and elbows relaxed and heavy.

5 Shift your weight back to the centre, and return to the *Horse Stance* with weight evenly distributed over both feet. Keep your arms in the same position. Shift your weight on to your right foot, and practise the movement on the right side. Repeat 4–5 times on each side, then return to the *Horse Stance* with arms by your sides.

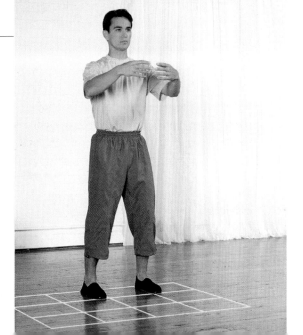

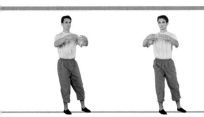

......Shift right......Turn right.....Repeat

BASIC BEAR

This is the most common tai chi warm-up exercise. Here you practise simultaneously shifting your weight and turning into the *Tai Chi Fold* as your arms move in a circular motion. Keep your arms relaxed to feel the momentum of the circular movement.

BENEFITS Increases hip flexibility; increases circulation to the hip joint, which tends to have a poor blood supply.

TIP Imagine that your head and torso are an upright column rotating over stable legs.

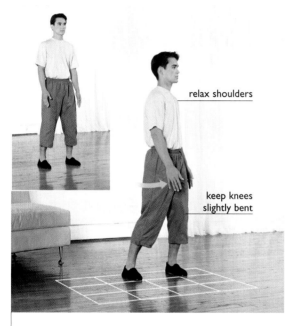

relax shoulders

keep knees slightly bent

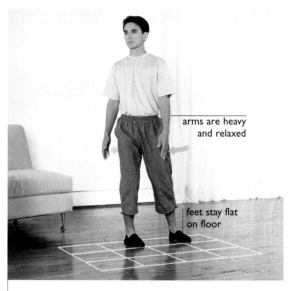

arms are heavy and relaxed

feet stay flat on floor

1 Stand in the *Horse Stance* with feet hip-width apart, knees slightly bent, and arms relaxed by your sides. Fold to the left by turning your pelvis and torso to the left as you shift your weight entirely on to your left foot. Simultaneously allow you arms to swing in a circular motion to the left with the movement of your pelvis and torso.

2 Fold to the right by turning your pelvis and torso to the right as you shift your weight entirely on to your right foot. Simultaneously swing your arms in a circular motion to the right with the movement of your pelvis and torso. Repeat the movement 7–8 times, then return to the *Horse Stance* with arms by your sides.

At a glance

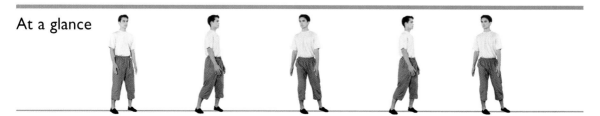

Arms by sides....Circle left...Circle right...Circle left...Circle right...Repeat

WALKING SKATING

Like the Basic Bear, this exercise involves "folding" and "sinking" into the weight-bearing leg in a natural, flowing sequence. The spiralling down and springing movement is similar to the action of throwing a ball.

> **BENEFITS** Improves flexibility in the joints; improves coordination.
>
> **TIPS** Vary the pace – try this very slowly, then more quickly. To sense qi in the fingertips, keep your shoulders relaxed and arms heavy.

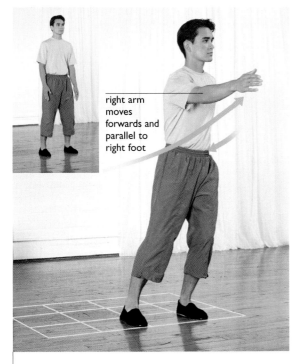

right arm moves forwards and parallel to right foot

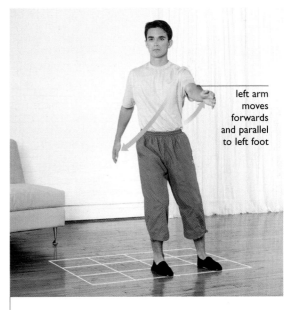

left arm moves forwards and parallel to left foot

1 Stand in the *Horse Stance* with feet hip-width apart, knees soft, and arms relaxed by your sides. Fold to the left by turning your pelvis and torso to the left as you shift your weight entirely on to your left foot. Simultaneously, swing your left arm back and your right arm forwards.

2 Fold to the right by turning your pelvis and torso to the right as you shift your weight entirely on to your right foot. Simultaneously swing your right arm back and left arm forwards. Repeat the movement 7–8 times, then return to the *Horse Stance* with arms by your sides.

At a glance

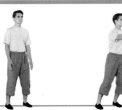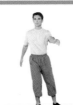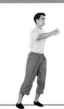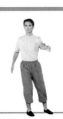

Arms by sides...Swing front...Swing back...Swing front...Swing back...Repeat

STEPPING BACK WITH THE FOLD

Folding and shifting on to the back foot creates a spiralling action that in martial arts is used to retreat while facing an opponent. Take small steps back to avoid arching your back and to ensure that you maintain a good centre of balance.

> **BENEFITS** Increases ankle flexibility; lengthens calf muscles; increases hip flexibility.
>
> **TIP** As you step back, focus on the outside edge of your foot as this will help you to keep it flat.

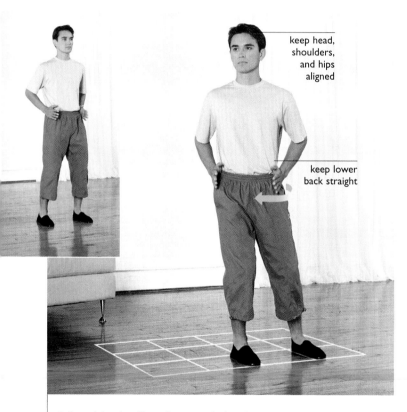

keep head, shoulders, and hips aligned

keep lower back straight

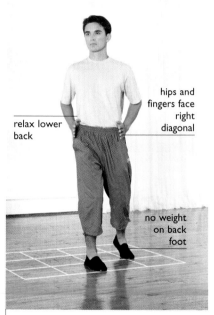

relax lower back

hips and fingers face right diagonal

no weight on back foot

1 Stand in the *Horse Stance* with feet hip-width apart, knees bent, and hands at your hips with fingers pointing forwards. Shift your weight entirely on to your right foot as you fold to the right by turning your pelvis and torso to the right.

2 Keeping all of your weight on your right foot, touch back on to the ball of your left foot.

At a glance

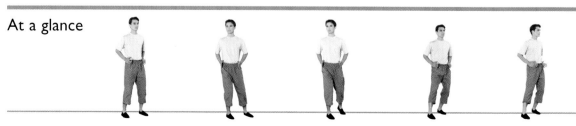

Weight centre....Fold right....Touch back......Shift/Turn......Fold left......

3 Transfer all of your weight on to your left foot, and turn your pelvis and torso so they face forwards.

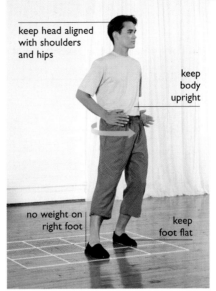

keep head aligned with shoulders and hips

keep body upright

no weight on right foot

keep foot flat

4 Keeping all of your weight on your left foot, fold to the left by turning your pelvis and torso to the left.

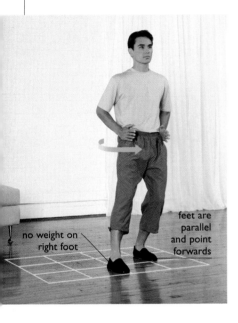

no weight on right foot

feet are parallel and point forwards

5 With your weight still on your left foot, step back, toes first, with your right foot.

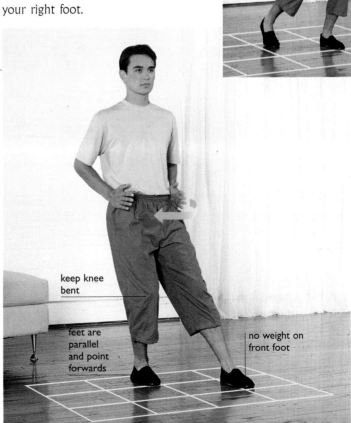

6 Shift your weight entirely on to your right foot as you turn your pelvis and torso to face forwards. Continue stepping back and folding 3–4 times or until comfortable with the footwork. Finally, return to the *Horse Stance* with arms by your sides.

keep knee bent

feet are parallel and point forwards

no weight on front foot

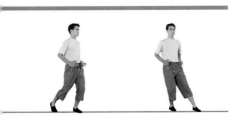

SIDE STEPPING WITH THE FOLD

This transitional movement teaches you to move sideways while maintaining a stable base. Remember to keep your feet flat on the floor and parallel throughout.

BENEFITS Strengthens muscles on the outer side of the hips and legs; increases strength and flexibility of the ankles.

TIPS To help keep feet flat, focus on the outside edge of your foot as you step; practise sliding your feet to the sides.

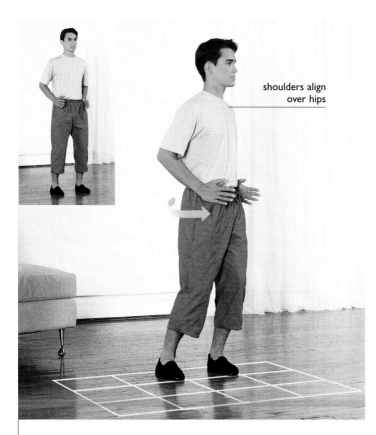

shoulders align over hips

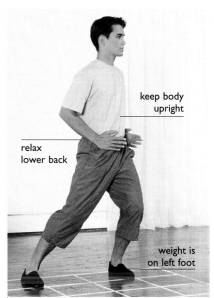

keep body upright

relax lower back

weight is on left foot

1 Stand in the *Horse Stance* with feet hip-width apart, knees bent, and hands at your hips. Shift your weight entirely on to your left foot as you fold to the left by turning your pelvis and torso to the left.

2 Step sideways with your right foot so that your feet are still parallel but are wider than hip-width apart. Stay folded to the left.

At a glance

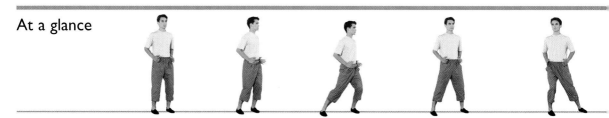

Weight centre.....Fold left.....Step sideways...Shift centre.....Fold right

3 Shift your weight to the centre as you turn your pelvis and torso to face forwards.

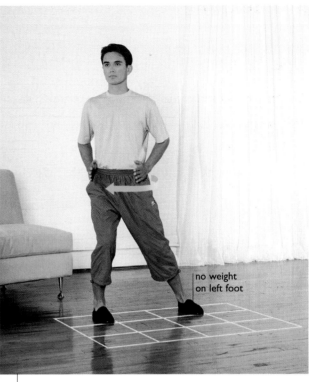

no weight
on left foot

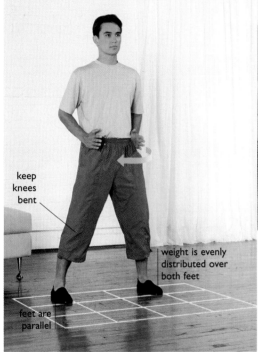

keep
knees
bent

weight is evenly
distributed over
both feet

feet are
parallel

4 Shift your weight entirely on to your right foot as you fold to the right by turning your pelvis and torso to the right.

5 Remain folded to the right, and move your left foot in closer so your feet are parallel and about hip-width apart. Then shift your weight back to the centre as you turn your pelvis and torso to face forwards. Repeat 3–4 times or more, then practise stepping to the right. Finally, return to the *Horse Stance* with arms by your sides.

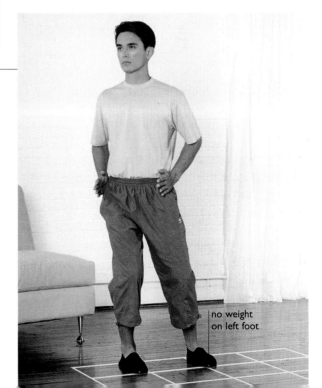

no weight
on left foot

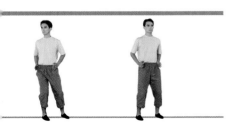

. . . . Step in . . . . Turn centre

HORSE STANCE TO TAI CHI STANCE

Here, the *Tai Chi Fold* is used to change direction and manoeuvre between two classic tai chi stances. As you "fold" and "sink" into your weighted leg, feel the spiralling action generate the turning of your torso. Keep both knees bent throughout the movement.

BENEFITS Good practice in maintaining body alignment and balance when moving into the *Tai Chi Fold* (pp54–55).

TIPS Relax; breathe slowly and deeply; keep your body upright and your pelvis relaxed; practise combining this move with *Tai Chi Stance to Horse Stance* (pp80–81).

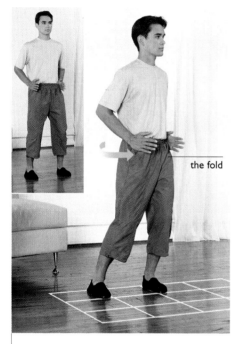

the fold

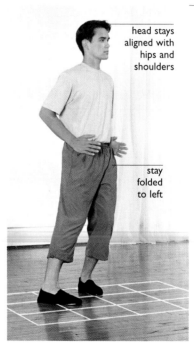

head stays aligned with hips and shoulders

stay folded to left

2 Keeping your weight entirely on your left foot, step forwards with your right foot so that it points diagonally inwards at a 45° angle.

1 Stand in the *Horse Stance* with feet hip-width apart, knees bent, and hands at your hips with fingers pointing forwards. Then shift your weight entirely on to your left foot as you fold to the left by turning your pelvis and torso to the left.

At a glance

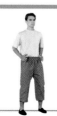 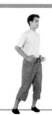 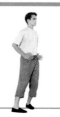 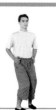 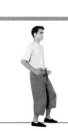

Weight centre......Fold left......Step forwards...Fold right.....Turn centre

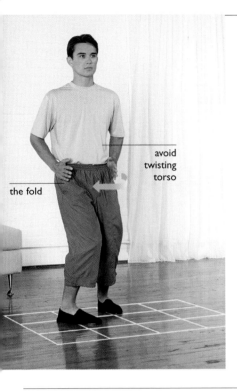

the fold

avoid
twisting
torso

3 Shift your weight entirely on to your right foot as you fold your pelvis and torso to the right.

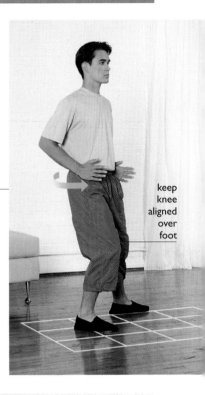

keep
knee
aligned
over
foot

4 Keeping your weight entirely on your right foot, turn your pelvis and torso to face the same direction as your right foot as you pivot on the ball of your left foot. Then step forwards with your left foot into the *Tai Chi Stance, Back Position.*

5 Shift 70 percent of your weight forwards on to your front, left foot. As you do this, turn your pelvis and torso to face forwards in the direction of your left foot to move into the *Tai Chi Stance, Forward Position.* Repeat 3–4 times or until you feel comfortable with the sequence. Then practise on the other side, beginning by folding to the right. Finally, move your feet parallel and relax.

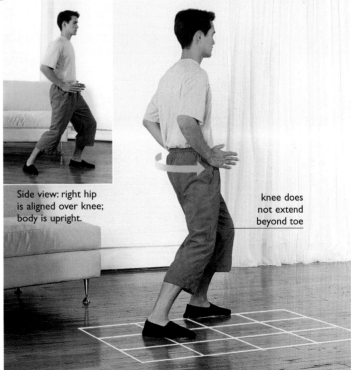

Side view: right hip
is aligned over knee;
body is upright.

knee does
not extend
beyond toe

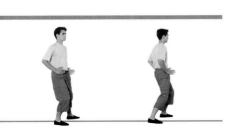

..Step forwards...Shift/Turn

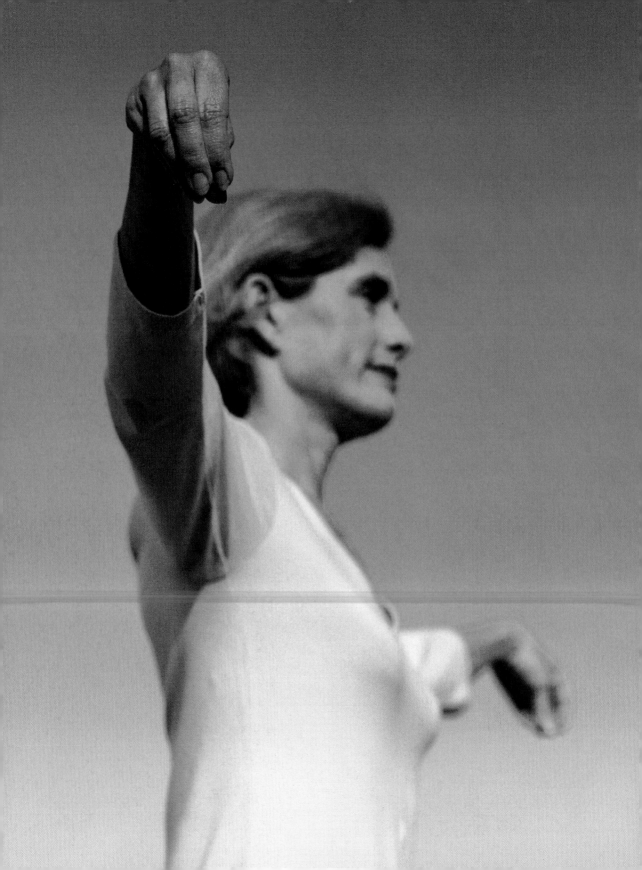

BASIC MOVES

PART THREE

These movements build on the skills learned in Parts One and Two and are the most advanced in terms of balance and coordination. They introduce the more complex movement patterns taught in Part Three of the Form. Here you move with open, expansive arms while balancing on one leg, and explore movement from the wide, stable stances of tai chi. Practise being simultaneously rooted, flexible, and free-flowing. Remember that you can work through the three parts of the Basic Moves and use them as a flowing exercise routine on their own.

HIGH STEP

In martial arts, the knee is raised to strike in this move. Practise holding your knee in the lifted position for as long as you can, then switch to the other leg. Remember to keep your shoulders and hips level throughout the movement.

BENEFITS Improves balance; increases thigh strength because knees are bent; increases hip and ankle flexibility and calf strength.

TIP Practise relaxing your legs: stand up, place both hands under your thigh, and lift it and hold it. Then let it drop.

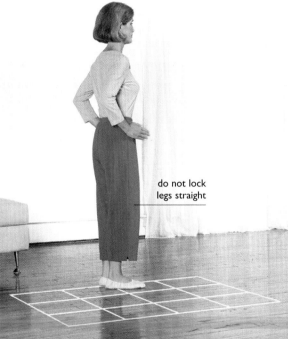

do not lock legs straight

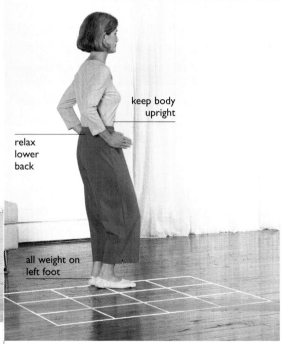

keep body upright

relax lower back

all weight on left foot

1 Stand straight with your heels close and your toes pointing outwards in a "V" shape. Keep your knees soft. Place your hands at your hips.

2 Bend your knees, and shift your weight entirely on to your left foot as you raise your right heel slightly off the ground.

At a glance

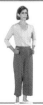   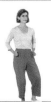 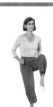

Weight centre.....Shift left...Raise knee...Lower knee..Shift right..Raise knee

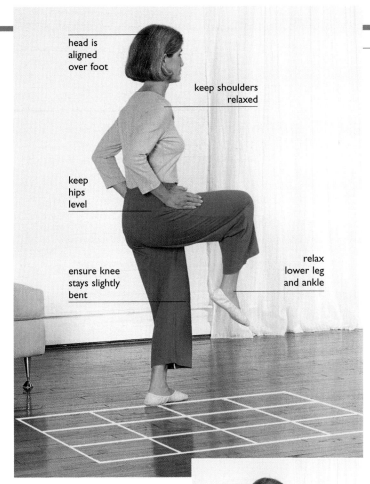

head is
aligned
over foot

keep shoulders
relaxed

keep
hips
level

ensure knee
stays slightly
bent

relax
lower leg
and ankle

3 Raise your right knee to about hip-height in front of you, keeping your lower leg and ankle relaxed – your lower leg should dangle from your knee. If you have trouble balancing, lower your right leg so that your toes touch the ground to steady you.

POINTS TO WATCH

• **Stand straight** – don't lean back, to the side, or raise one hip as this will affect your balance.

• **Keep** your standing leg bent to avoid straining the knee.

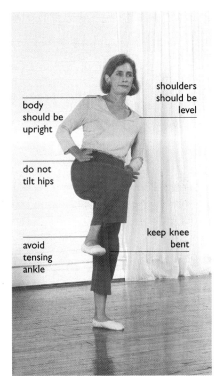

shoulders
should be
level

body
should be
upright

do not
tilt hips

avoid
tensing
ankle

keep knee
bent

4 Slowly lower your right leg and return your foot to the "V"-shape starting position. Then shift your weight on to your right foot and repeat on the other side. Repeat the movement 3–4 times on each leg, then return to the start position.

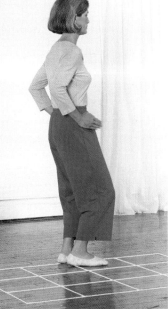

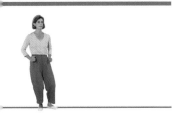

.....L o w e r   k n e e . . R e p e a t

FLYING CRANE

This graceful movement involves balancing on one foot in a continuous weight-shifting pattern. It is the *High Step* combined with arm movements similar to *Crane Takes Flight*. The key is to maintain stability and a sense of flow throughout the movement, especially as you shift your weight on to your standing leg. Practise coordinating your breathing with your arm movements.

BENEFITS Improves shoulder flexibility and arm strength; enhances coordination; coordinating breathing and relaxed movement enhances flow of qi.

TIP Imagine that you are a graceful crane flying high above the clouds.

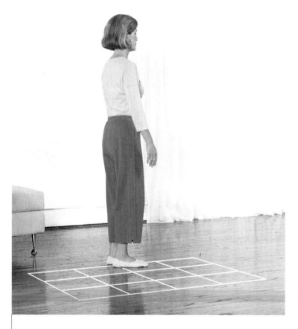

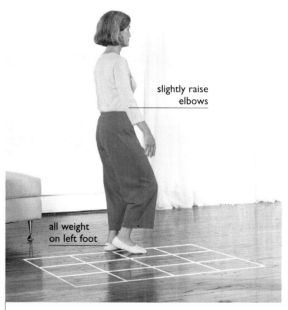

slightly raise elbows

all weight on left foot

1 Stand straight with your heels close and your toes pointing outwards in a "V" shape. Keep your knees soft, and relax your arms at your sides. Breathe slowly and deeply.

2 Exhale as you bend your knees, shift your weight entirely on to your left foot, and raise your right heel slightly off the ground. Simultaneously begin to raise your elbows at your sides.

At a glance

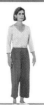   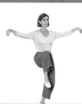 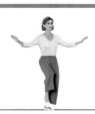

Breathe naturally...Exhale.........Inhale to raise arms ....Exhale to

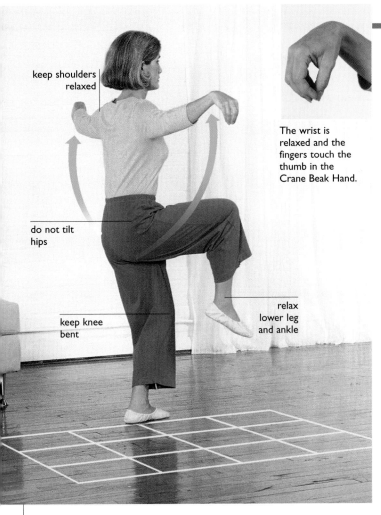

keep shoulders
relaxed

do not tilt
hips

keep knee
bent

relax
lower leg
and ankle

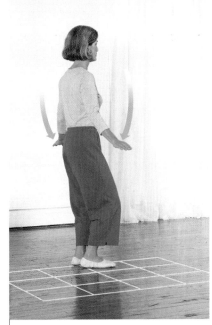

The wrist is
relaxed and the
fingers touch the
thumb in the
Crane Beak Hand.

3 Raise your right knee to about hip-height in front of you, keeping your lower leg and ankle relaxed. Inhale as you raise your arms to shoulder-height at your sides, leading with your wrists and forming the *Crane Beak Hand*. If you have trouble balancing, lower your right leg so that your toes touch the ground to steady you.

4 Slowly lower your right foot to the starting position as you exhale and lower your arms, leading with your wrists. Then shift your weight on to your right foot and repeat on the other side. Repeat the movement 3–4 times on each leg, then return to the start position.

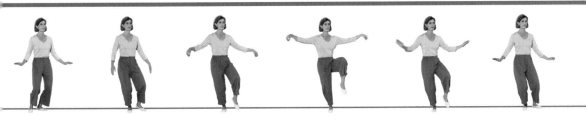

l o w e r   a r m s . . . . I n h a l e   t o   r a i s e   a r m s . . . . . E x h a l e   t o   l o w e r   a r m s . . . . . R e p e a t

TOE KICK

This kick to the diagonal requires leg strength and flexibility at the hip joint. As you kick, raise your leg and foot in one movement. Practise holding this position for as long as you can. Take care to keep your hips straight throughout the movement.

> **BENEFITS** Increases flexibility in hip and groin muscles; improves balance; increases leg and hip strength.
>
> **TIP** If you have trouble balancing, use a wall or stable chair for support. Alternatively, lower your kicking leg so that your toes touch the ground to steady you.

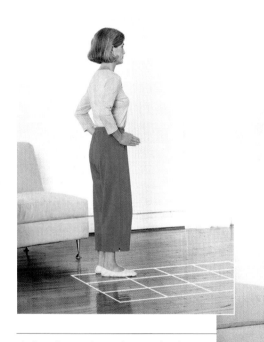

1 Stand straight with your heels close and your toes pointing outwards in a "V" shape. Keep your knees soft, and place your hands at your hips. Then bend your knees and shift your weight entirely on to your left foot.

raise right heel slightly off ground

At a glance

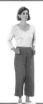 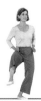 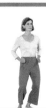

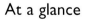
Weight centre..........Shift left............Raise leg...........Lower leg.......

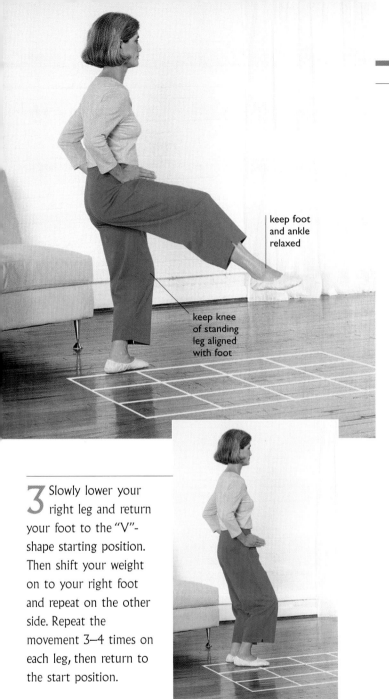

keep foot
and ankle
relaxed

keep knee
of standing
leg aligned
with foot

2 Keeping your left knee bent, lift your right foot to the right diagonal with knee hip-height and ankle relaxed. Keep your body upright and ensure that your hips stay straight and facing forwards. If you have trouble balancing, lower your right leg so that your toes touch the ground to steady you.

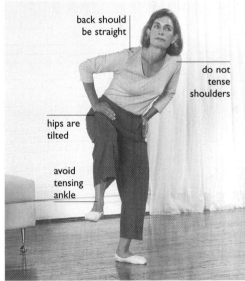

back should
be straight

do not
tense
shoulders

hips are
tilted

avoid
tensing
ankle

3 Slowly lower your right leg and return your foot to the "V"-shape starting position. Then shift your weight on to your right foot and repeat on the other side. Repeat the movement 3–4 times on each leg, then return to the start position.

POINTS TO WATCH

- **Keep** your body upright, head, shoulders, and hips aligned, and back straight. Use your hands to help you check the position of your hips.
- **Do not** lean forwards.
- **Relax** your neck and shoulders
- **Do not** tilt your head.
- **Relax** your lower leg and ankle of your kicking leg.

..Shift right.........Raise leg......Lower leg....Repeat

DANCING CRANE

This expressive exercise combines the *Toe Kick* with the arm movements from *Gathering the Stars*. Practise holding the start and end positions, then combine the movements in a continuous flow.

BENEFITS Opens the chest and improves posture; enhances balance; arm movements add a cardiovascular benefit; coordinating movement with breathing can have an emotionally uplifting effect.

TIPS Coordinate your breathing with the movement: inhale when expanding, exhale when gathering. Focus on your palms and fingertips as you open and close your arms as this enhances the flow of qi in the body.

keep shoulders relaxed

relax elbows

keep lower back relaxed

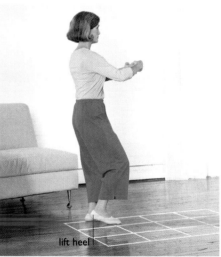

lift heel

1 Stand straight with your heels close and your toes pointing outwards in a "V" shape. Keep your knees soft. Raise your arms in front of you as if holding a large ball, with your fingers and thumbs facing each other, in the *Holding the Moon Position* (*see p23*). Breathe slowly and deeply.

2 As you exhale, bend your knees and shift your weight entirely on to your left foot.

At a glance

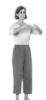   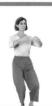

Breathe naturally...Exhale....Inhale to open............Exhale to close.........

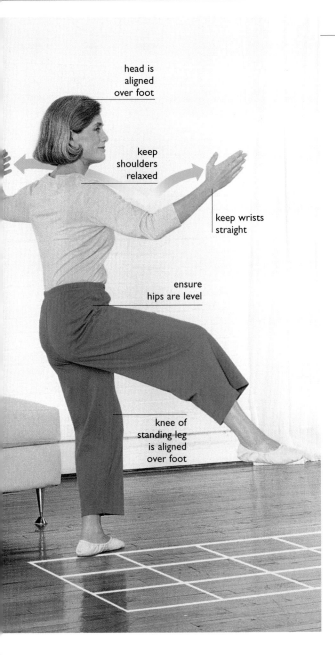

head is
aligned
over foot

keep
shoulders
relaxed

keep wrists
straight

ensure
hips are level

knee of
standing leg
is aligned
over foot

3 Keeping your left knee bent, inhale as you raise your right foot to the right diagonal, with knee hip-height and ankle relaxed. At the same time, open your arms and turn your head slightly as you gaze to the right. If you have trouble balancing, lower your right knee so that your toes touch the ground to steady you.

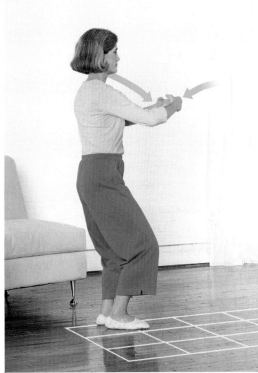

4 Slowly lower your right leg and return your foot to the "V"-shape start position as you exhale and bring your arms back to the *Holding the Moon Position.* Then shift your weight on to your right foot and repeat on the other side. Repeat 3–4 times on each side, then return to the start position.

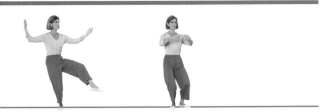

...Inhale to open.....Exhale to close....Repeat

THE TAI CHI STANCE WITH FOLD

Here, you learn to combine the stable base of the *Tai Chi Stance* with the wind-up motion of the *Tai Chi Fold*, a characteristic pattern of tai chi movement. The move involves shifting your weight as you simultaneously turn your pelvis and torso.

BENEFITS Same as *Tai Chi Stance (pp46–47)* and *Tai Chi Fold (pp54–55)*. Increases flexibility and strength in hips and legs; improves balance in a wide stance.

TIP Keep knees bent and remain at the same height throughout the movement.

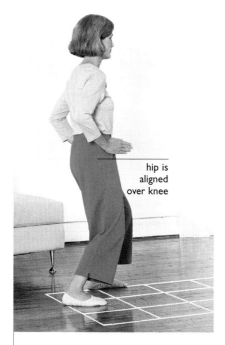

hip is aligned over knee

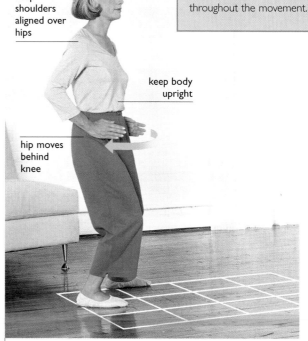

keep shoulders aligned over hips

keep body upright

hip moves behind knee

1 Stand in the *Tai Chi Stance, Forward Position*, with your left foot forward supporting 70 percent of your weight and your right foot back and turned outwards at a 45° angle. Your pelvis faces the direction of your front foot. Place your hands at your hips.

2 Shift all of your weight back on to your right foot as you simultaneously fold to the right by turning your pelvis and torso towards the back, right leg. This is the *Tai Chi Stance with Fold*.

At a glance

 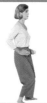 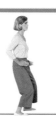 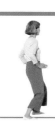

Weight forward..........Fold right......Align knee.......Shift/Turn...Repeat

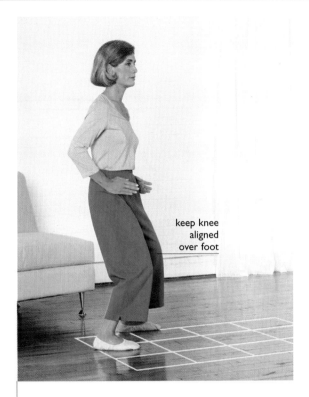

keep knee
aligned
over foot

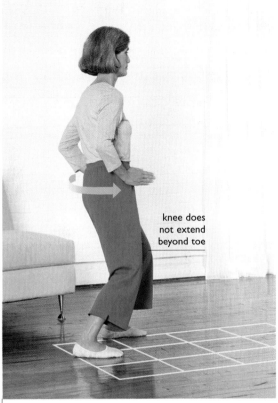

knee does
not extend
beyond toe

3 Bend your left knee, aligning it over the centre of your left foot. Remember to relax your hip joint as you feel your weight sink into your left foot.

4 Shift 70 percent of your weight forwards on to your left foot as you simultaneously turn your pelvis and torso to face forwards in the direction of the front leg to move into the *Tai Chi Stance, Forward Position*. Repeat 3–4 times, or until you feel comfortable with the move. Then practise starting with your right foot forward. Finally, move feet parallel and relax.

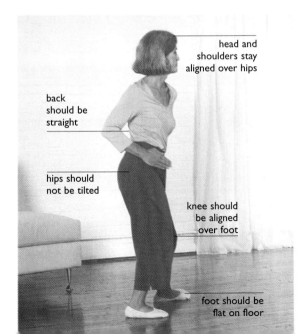

head and
shoulders stay
aligned over hips

back
should be
straight

hips should
not be tilted

knee should
be aligned
over foot

foot should be
flat on floor

POINTS TO WATCH

- **Move** your torso and pelvis as a unit – don't lead with the shoulders or twist the torso.
- **Keep** your body upright, and avoid arching the back.
- **Avoid** tilting your hips; keep them level.
- **Keep** your front knee aligned over the centre of your foot; otherwise, you put strain on the knee.

THE TAI CHI POWER MOVE

This move provides optimal power with minimal effort. Shifting back and turning produces a wind-up motion that generates the forward arm movement. Practise the *Basic Bear* and *Walking Skating* to perfect the arm movements.

BENEFITS Excellent for improving coordination; arm movements increase hip flexibility.

TIPS *The Tai Chi Classics* says "The motion should be rooted in the feet, released through the legs, guided by the torso, and expressed through the fingers." Imagine throwing a ball underhand.

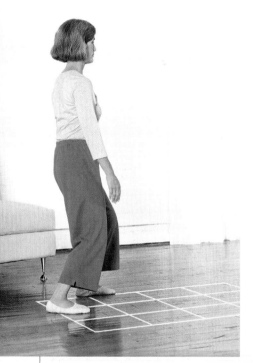

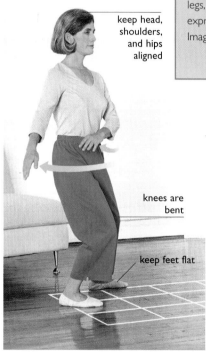

keep head, shoulders, and hips aligned

knees are bent

keep feet flat

1 Stand in the *Tai Chi Stance, Forward Position,* with your left foot forward supporting 70 percent of your weight and your right foot back and turned outwards at a 45° angle. Your pelvis faces the direction of your front foot. Relax your arms at your sides.

2 Shift all of your weight back on to your right foot and turn your pelvis and torso towards the back, right leg into the *Tai Chi Stance* with the *Fold.* As you do this, allow your left arm to swing in a circular motion in front of your body (to the right) as your right arm swings back in a wind-up motion as if preparing to pitch a ball underhand or roll a bowling ball.

At a glance

  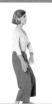 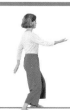

Arms at sides...Circle and swing right...Circle and swing forwards..Repeat

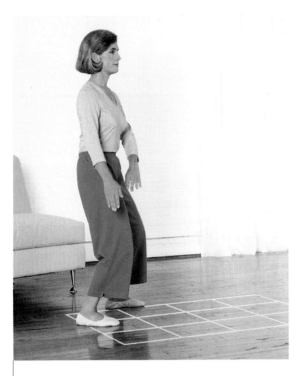

3 Bend your left knee, aligning it over the centre of the left foot, as you begin to swing your right arm forwards.

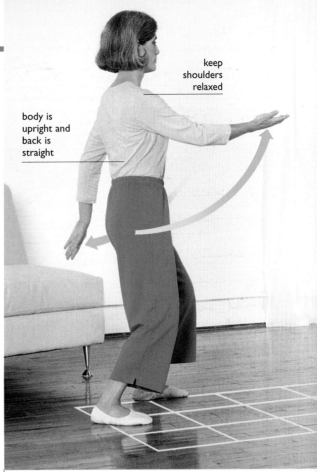

keep shoulders relaxed

body is upright and back is straight

4 Shift 70 percent of your weight forwards on to your left foot and simultaneously rotate your pelvis and torso to face forwards in the direction of the front leg to move into the *Tai Chi Stance, Forward Position.* As you do this, swing your right arm forwards and your left arm back. Repeat 3–4 times, or until you feel comfortable with the movement, then practise with your right root forward. Finally, move feet parallel and relax.

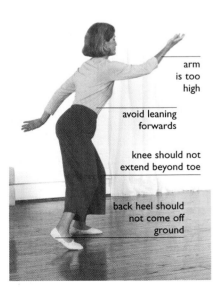

arm is too high

avoid leaning forwards

knee should not extend beyond toe

back heel should not come off ground

POINTS TO WATCH

• **Do not** lean forwards or arch your back.

• **Both feet** remain flat on the ground to create a stable base.

• **Relax** your arms as you swing them, and stay within your natural range of motion – don't reach forwards.

TAI CHI STANCE TO HORSE STANCE

This essential transitional move teaches you how to change direction when moving between these two classical tai chi stances. Remember to keep your body upright at all times and to use your hands to guide the correct positioning of the pelvis and torso.

BENEFITS Increases flexibility and strength in the hips and legs; improves balance and coordination; turning foot inwards improves ankle and calf flexibility.

TIP Practise combining this move with *Horse Stance to Tai Chi Stance* (*pp64–65*).

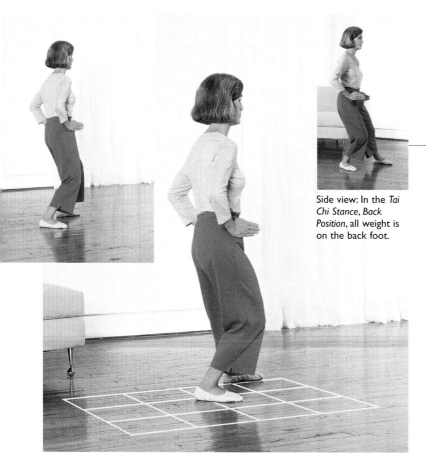

Side view: In the *Tai Chi Stance, Back Position*, all weight is on the back foot.

1 Stand with 70 percent of your weight on your left, front foot, in the *Tai Chi Stance, Forward Position*, and place your hands at your hips. Then move into the *Tai Chi Stance, Back Position*, by shifting all of your weight on to your back, right foot.

At a glance

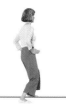 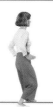 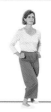 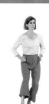

Weight forward..........Shift back..........Fold right.......Pivot forwards.......

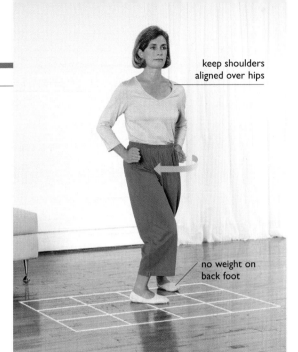
keep shoulders
aligned over hips

no weight on
back foot

2 With all of your weight on the right foot, fold
to the right by turning your pelvis and torso to
the right. Simultaneously turn your left leg and foot
90° inwards to the right, pivoting on your heel.

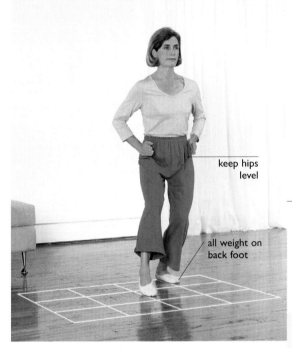
keep hips
level

all weight on
back foot

3 Shift all of your weight on to your
left foot, pivoting on the toes of
your right foot so that your pelvis, torso,
and both feet face forwards.

4 Keeping your weight on your left foot, step
back with your right foot so that your feet
are parallel and about hip-width apart. Then shift
your weight to the centre and move into the
Horse Stance. Repeat 3–4 times, or until you feel
comfortable with the sequence. Then practise
starting with your right foot forward, finally ending
in the Horse Stance with your arms by your sides.

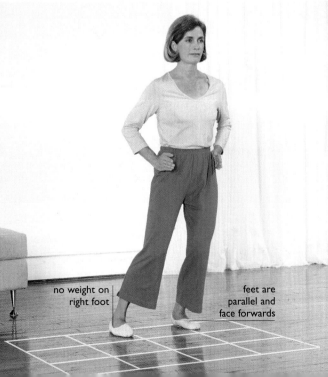
no weight on
right foot

feet are
parallel and
face forwards

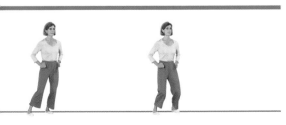

...Step back........Shift centre......Repeat

BASIC MOVES SUMMARY

Use this summary as a reference for all of the basic moves presented in this book. Once you are familiar with them, refer to this summary to remind you of the order of the moves in each section and for practising the entire sequence. Remember to warm up (*see pp24–29*) and to practise sensing qi (*see pp20–23*) before each session. You may want to finish with the exercises for moving and gathering qi (*see pp148–153*).

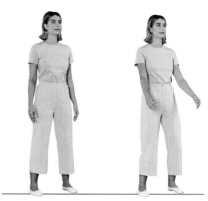

Horse stance
p34

Heavy arms
p35

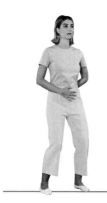
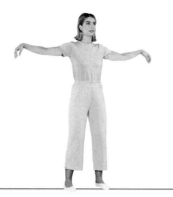
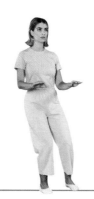
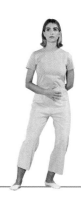

Riding the horse
pp36–37

Crane takes flight
pp38–39

Bear roots on one leg
pp40–41

Stable and open
pp42–43

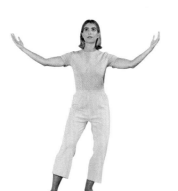
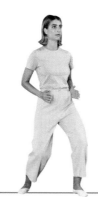
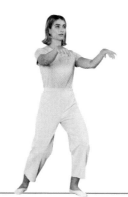
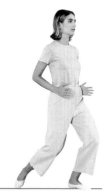

Gathering the stars
pp44–45

The tai chi stance
pp46–47

Bear moves with
crane arms
pp48–49

Tai chi stance
forward transition
pp50–51

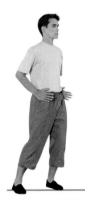
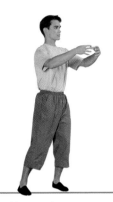
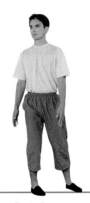
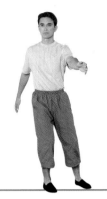
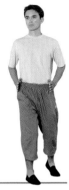

The tai chi fold
pp54–55

Moving the moon
pp56–57

Basic bear
p58

Walking skating
p59

Stepping back
with the fold
pp60–61

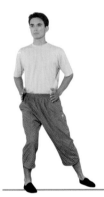
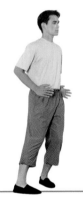
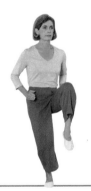
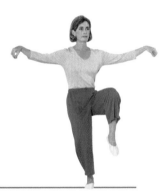

Stepping sideways
with the fold
pp62–63

Horse stance to tai
chi stance
pp64–65

High step
pp68–69

Flying crane
pp70–71

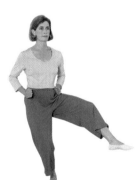
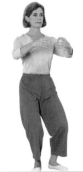
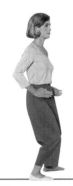
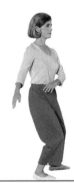
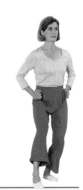

Toe Kick
pp72–73

Dancing crane
pp74–75

The tai chi stance
with the fold
pp76–77

The tai chi
power move
pp78–79

Tai chi stance to
horse stance
pp80–81

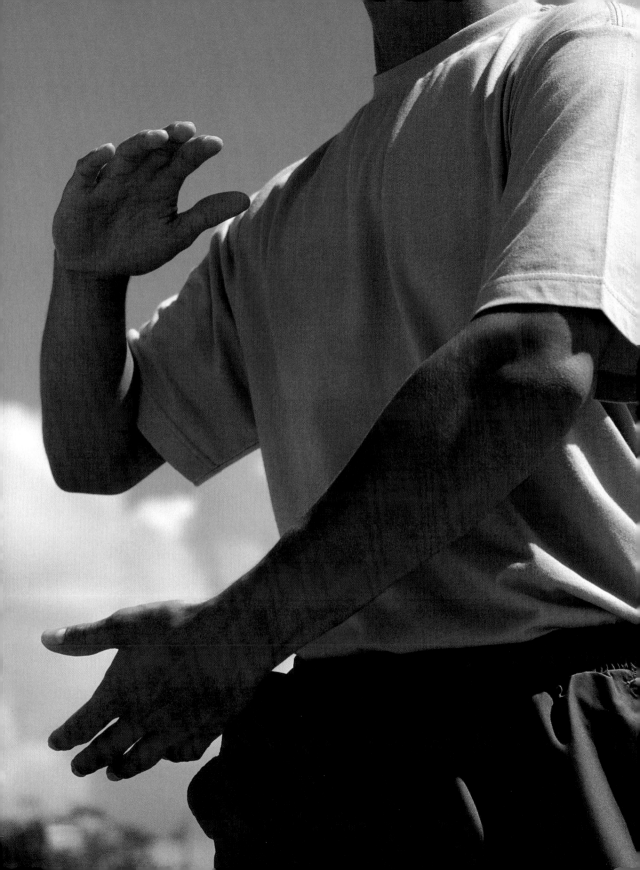

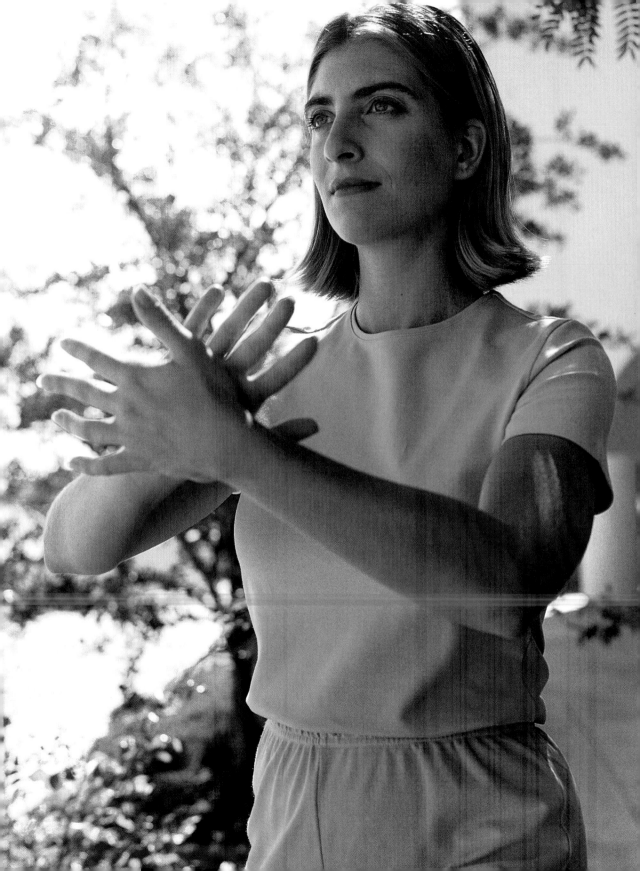

THE
FORM

This form lays the groundwork for all Yang-Style tai chi. It is divided into three parts. As you progress, the movements become more complex, building on what you have learnt before. Relax and maintain awareness of your breathing as you move. Eventually your movements and breathing will naturally coordinate. As you practise the Form, refer back to the Basic Moves to ensure you maintain correct technique. Practise sensing qi and breathing (*see pp18–23*), and warm up (*see pp24–29*) before you begin.

PART ONE

This part introduces the basic stances and forward transitions of the tai chi Form. Before you begin, stand quietly for a few minutes and let your mind become as clear as the open sky. As you practise tai chi, consider the unity of all things.

PREPARATION

Imagine your starting point here to be the centre, or balance point, of the yin-yang symbol, or tai chi diagram. When practising tai chi, you are moving along the curved line where the opposites join, which represents the path of least resistance, or the "middle path". Review *Basic Moves: Horse Stance* (p34), *Stable and Open* (pp42–43).

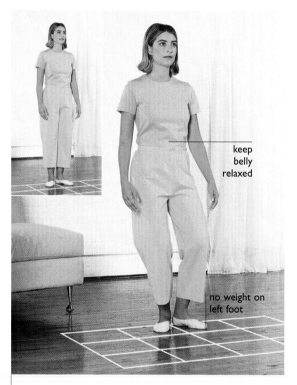

keep belly relaxed

no weight on left foot

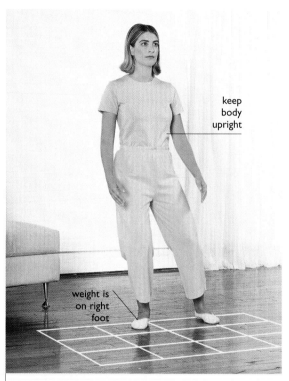

keep body upright

weight is on right foot

1 Stand with your body upright and relaxed and your feet in a "V" position with heels together at a 45° angle. Allow your arms to hang relaxed at your sides. Then shift your weight entirely on to your right foot.

2 Step to the side with your left foot so that it is hip-width from your right and pointing forwards.

At a glance

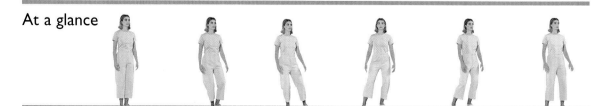

Weight centre...Shift right....Step left...Shift/Turn...Turn centre...Shift centre

3 Shift all of your weight on to your left foot, keeping your knee aligned over your foot, as you turn your pelvis and torso to the right diagonal. Simultaneously turn your palms to face each other.

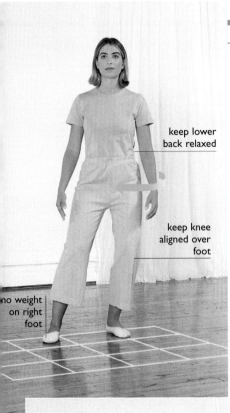

keep lower back relaxed

keep knee aligned over foot

no weight on right foot

4 Keeping your weight entirely on your left foot, turn your pelvis and torso back to the centre, pivoting on your right heel and bringing your right foot parallel to the left one.

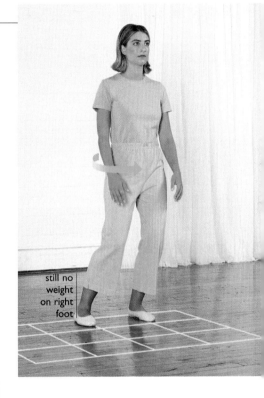

still no weight on right foot

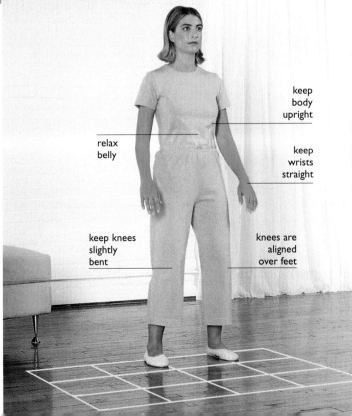

keep body upright

relax belly

keep wrists straight

keep knees slightly bent

knees are aligned over feet

5 Shift your weight to centre so that it is evenly distributed over both feet in the *Horse Stance.* Your feet are parallel and hip-width apart. Simultaneously move your arms so that they hang relaxed at your sides with your elbows slightly bent and wrists straight. Your fingers point down and forwards in the *Wu Chi Position.* To continue, move to *Beginning* (see over).

BEGINNING

As you raise your arms, imagine that your hands are moving through water, and focus on relaxing your wrists. Move like a river that flows slowly along its natural course. In the martial arts application, the arms are raised to strike and block. Review *Basic Moves: Horse Stance* (p34).

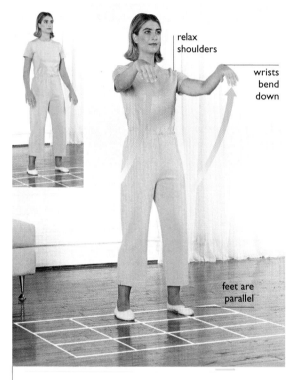

relax
shoulders

wrists
bend
down

feet are
parallel

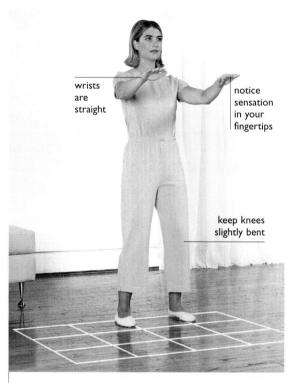

wrists
are
straight

notice
sensation
in your
fingertips

keep knees
slightly bent

1 Stand in the *Horse Stance* with feet hip-width apart and arms by your sides in the *Wu Chi Position*. Then raise your arms to shoulder height and width in front of you, keeping your wrists relaxed so that your fingers point downwards.

2 Bend your elbows slightly as you straighten your wrists and raise your hands so that your fingers point forwards and your palms face the floor.

At a glance

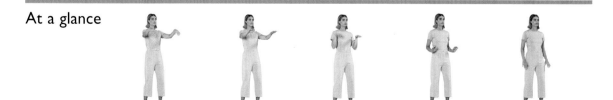

Raise arms...Raise hands...Bend elbows...Lower wrists...Raise hands

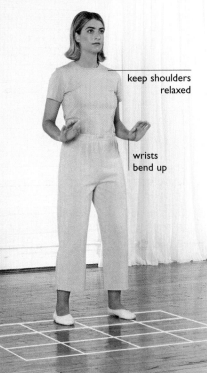

wrists
bend
down

leave space
between
body and
arms

3 Draw your hands towards your shoulders, bending your elbows and wrists. As you move your arms, keep your shoulders relaxed, your fingers pointing forwards, and your palms facing the floor.

keep shoulders
relaxed

wrists
bend up

4 Move your elbows back and, leading with your wrists, lower your hands to waist height with fingers pointing up and forwards.

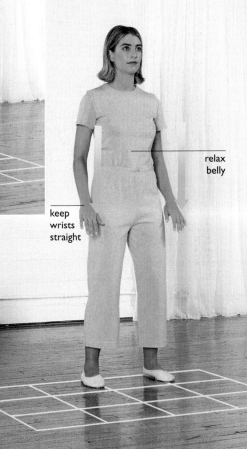

relax
belly

keep
wrists
straight

5 Slowly lower your fingers as your hands move just below hip height. Your arms are now in the *Wu Chi Position*, relaxed at your sides with your elbows slightly bent and wrists straight. Your fingers point down and forwards. To continue, move to *Ward Off (Left)* (see over).

WARD OFF (LEFT)

Imagine that you are catching a beach ball thrown to your right side. Then hold the ball between your left arm and your chest. The Tai Chi Classics say, "In motion, let all parts of the body be light, nimble and strung together." Review *Basic Moves: Horse Stance* (p34), *Stable and Open* (pp42–43), *Tai Chi Stance* (pp46–47).

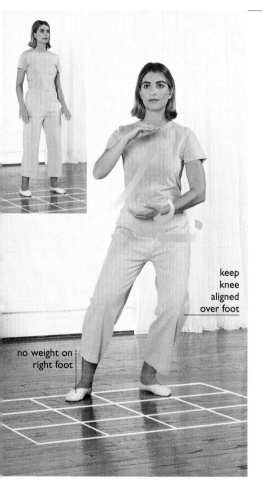

keep knee aligned over foot

no weight on right foot

1 From the *Horse Stance* with arms in the *Wu Chi Position*, shift your weight entirely on to your left foot as you turn your pelvis and torso to the right and pivot on your right heel to face the diagonal in the *Stable and Open Position*. Simultaneously move your right hand to chest height, facing down, and your left hand to belly height, facing up as if holding a large ball.

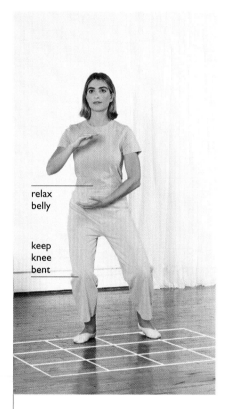

relax belly

keep knee bent

2 Shift your weight entirely on to your right foot, keeping your lower back relaxed. Maintain the same arm position.

At a glance

   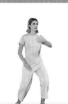

Shift/Turn.........Shift right.........Step forwards......Shift/Turn

3 Keeping your weight entirely on your right foot, step directly forwards with your left foot, feet hip-width apart, into the *Tai Chi Stance, Back Position.* Your arms still maintain the same position.

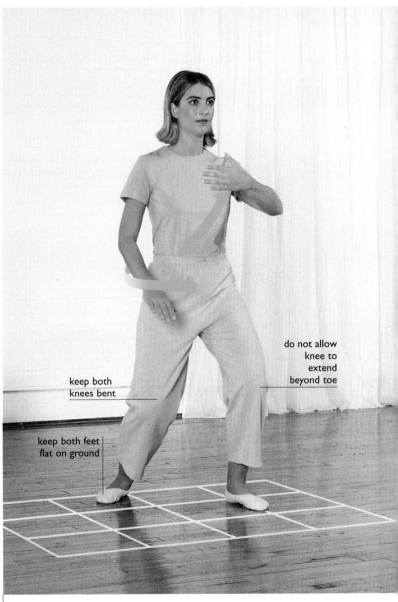

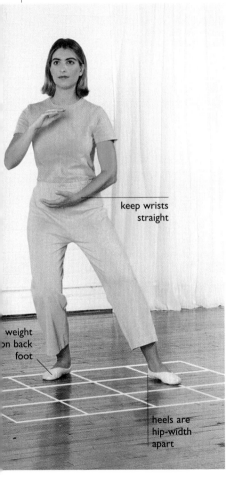

keep wrists straight

weight on back foot

heels are hip-width apart

do not allow knee to extend beyond toe

keep both knees bent

keep both feet flat on ground

4 Shift 70 percent of your weight forwards on to your left foot as you turn your pelvis and torso to face the direction of your left foot in the *Tai Chi Stance, Forward Position.* Simultaneously raise your left arm so that your palm faces your chest as you lower your right arm down next to your right hip with your elbow slightly bent and your fingers pointing down and slightly forwards. Your arms are in the *Ward Off Position.*
To continue, move to *Press (Left)* (see over).

PRESS (LEFT)

As you shift back, allow all of your weight to rest on your back foot. This provides a firmer stance and means that you cannot easily be thrown off balance. Review *Basic Moves: Bear Moves with Crane Arms* (pp48–49).

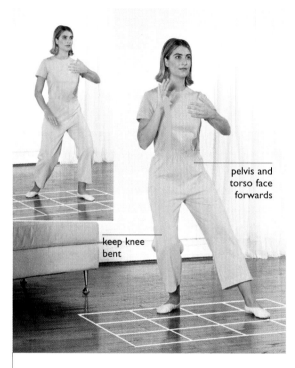

pelvis and torso face forwards

keep knee bent

1 From the *Tai Chi Stance, Forward Position*, arms in the *Ward Off Position*, shift all of your weight on to your back, right foot to move into the *Tai Chi Stance, Back Position*. As you shift back, bend your right elbow so that your palm faces forwards and fingers point up.

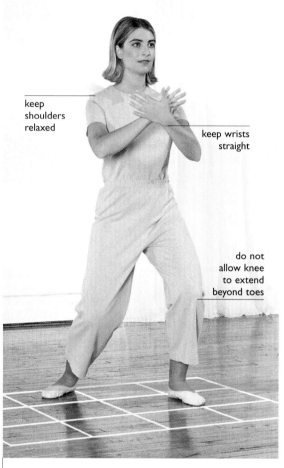

keep shoulders relaxed

keep wrists straight

do not allow knee to extend beyond toes

2 Shift 70 percent of your weight forwards on to your left, front foot to move into the *Tai Chi Stance, Forward Position*. Simultaneously move your arms into the *Press Position* by lowering your left elbow slightly so that your elbows are level, and pressing your right palm lightly into the wrist and base of your left palm.

At a glance

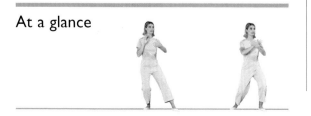

Shift back..Shift forwards

PUSH (LEFT)

As you shift back, imagine that your arms move behind and slightly under a large ball. As you shift forwards, keep your arms relaxed. The power comes from your legs. Review *Basic Moves: Bear Moves with Crane Arms* **(pp48–49)**.

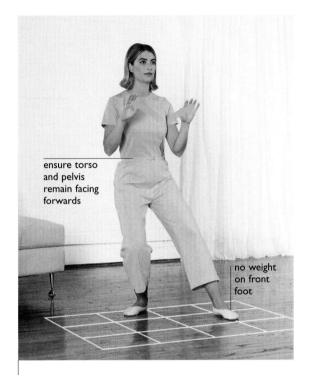

ensure torso
and pelvis
remain facing
forwards

no weight
on front
foot

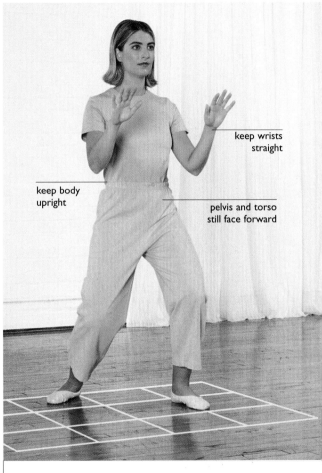

keep wrists
straight

keep body
upright

pelvis and torso
still face forward

1 Shift your weight entirely on to your right, back foot to move into the *Tai Chi Stance, Back Position*. As you shift back, move your arms into the *Push Position* by lowering both elbows so that your forearms are parallel to each other in front of you, both palms at chest height facing forwards and slightly down.

2 Shift 70 percent of your weight forwards on to your left foot to move into the *Tai Chi Stance, Forward Position*. Keep your arms in the *Push Position*, but swing your elbows forwards slightly. To continue, move to *Ward Off (Right)* (see over).

At a glance

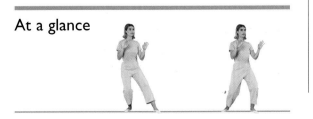

Shift back.......Shift forwards

WARD OFF (RIGHT)

Imagine that your right wrist is being lifted by a string as it blocks and strikes in the *Ward Off*. Practise with a peaceful, quiet mind. Concentrate on moving slowly and precisely, and remain focused on the moment. Review *Basic Moves: Tai Chi Stance, Forward Transition* (pp50–51).

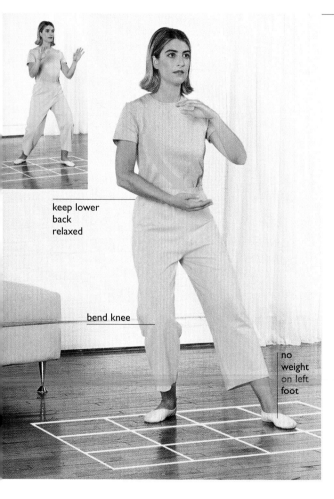

keep lower back relaxed

bend knee

no weight on left foot

1 From the *Tai Chi Stance, Forward Position*, arms in the *Push Position*, shift all of your weight on to your right, back foot to move into the *Tai Chi Stance, Back Position*. Simultaneously move your left hand so that your palm faces down, and lower your right hand to belly height, palm facing up as if holding a large ball.

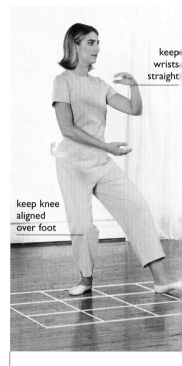

keep wrists straight

keep knee aligned over foot

2 Turn your pelvis and torso to the left, pivoting on your left heel to turn your left foot diagonally outwards. Your arms remain in the same position.

At a glance

 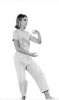 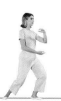 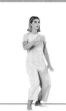

Shift back...Turn left....Shift left....Step forwards...Shift/Turn

3 Shift all of your weight on to your left foot to move into the *Forward Transition*.

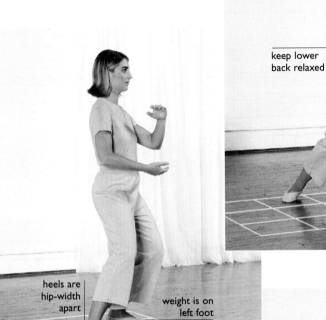

keep body upright

keep lower back relaxed

heels are hip-width apart

weight is on left foot

4 Step forwards with your right foot into the *Tai Chi Stance, Back Position*. Your arms remain in the same position.

5 Move into the *Tai Chi Stance, Forward Position* by shifting 70 percent of your weight forwards on to your right foot as you turn your pelvis and torso to face the direction of your right foot. Keep both knees bent. Simultaneously move your arms into the *Ward Off Position* by raising your right palm so that it faces your chest, and lowering your left arm down next to your left hip, keeping your elbow slightly bent, and your fingers pointing down and forwards. To continue, move to *Press (Right)* (see over).

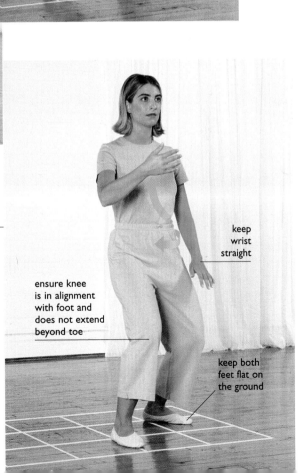

keep wrist straight

ensure knee is in alignment with foot and does not extend beyond toe

keep both feet flat on the ground

PRESS (RIGHT)

Press with a very light touch. As you press, feel the warmth of your left hand on your right wrist. Notice any changes in sensation in your palms and fingertips. Review *Basic Moves: Bear Moves with Crane Arms* (pp48–49).

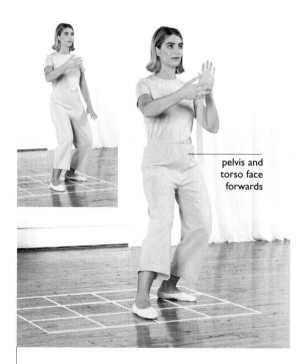

pelvis and
torso face
forwards

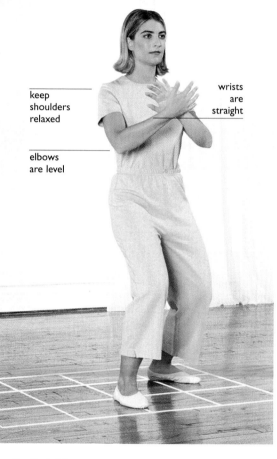

keep
shoulders
relaxed

wrists
are
straight

elbows
are level

1 From the *Tai Chi Stance, Forward Position*, arms in the *Ward Off Position*, shift your weight entirely on to your left, back foot to move into the *Tai Chi Stance, Back Position*. As you shift back, bend your left elbow and bring your hand up to chest height, palm facing forwards.

2 Shift 70 percent of your weight forwards on to your right, front foot to move into the *Tai Chi Stance, Forward Position*. Simultaneously, lower your right elbow slightly, and press your left palm lightly into the wrist and base of your right palm so that your arms are in the *Press Position*.

At a glance

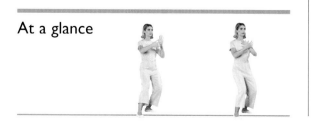

Shift back..Shift forwards

PUSH (RIGHT)

As you shift back, sink your shoulders and elbows down. Imagine that you are pushing the surface of a large ball that is clearing obstacles in front of you. *Basic Moves: Bear Moves with Crane Arms* **(pp48–49).**

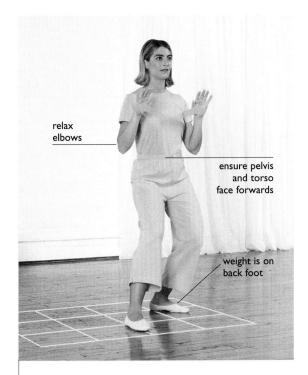

relax elbows

ensure pelvis and torso face forwards

weight is on back foot

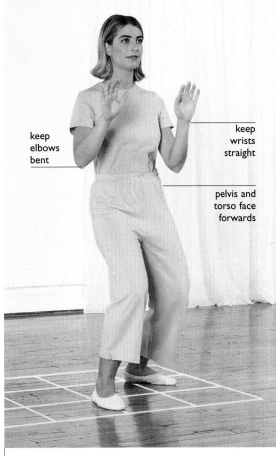

keep elbows bent

keep wrists straight

pelvis and torso face forwards

1 Shift your weight entirely on to your left, back foot to move into the *Tai Chi Stance, Back Position.* Simultaneously move your arms into the *Push Position* by lowering both elbows so that your forearms are parallel to each other in front of you, and both palms are at chest height facing forwards and slightly down.

2 Shift 70 percent of your weight forwards on to your right, front foot to move into the *Tai Chi Stance, Forward Position.* Keep your hands in the *Push Position,* but swing your elbows slightly forwards. Finish here, or, to continue, move to *Repulse Monkey, Arms* (pp102–103).

At a glance

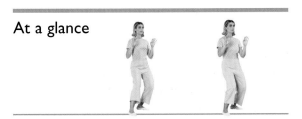

Shift back....Shift forwards

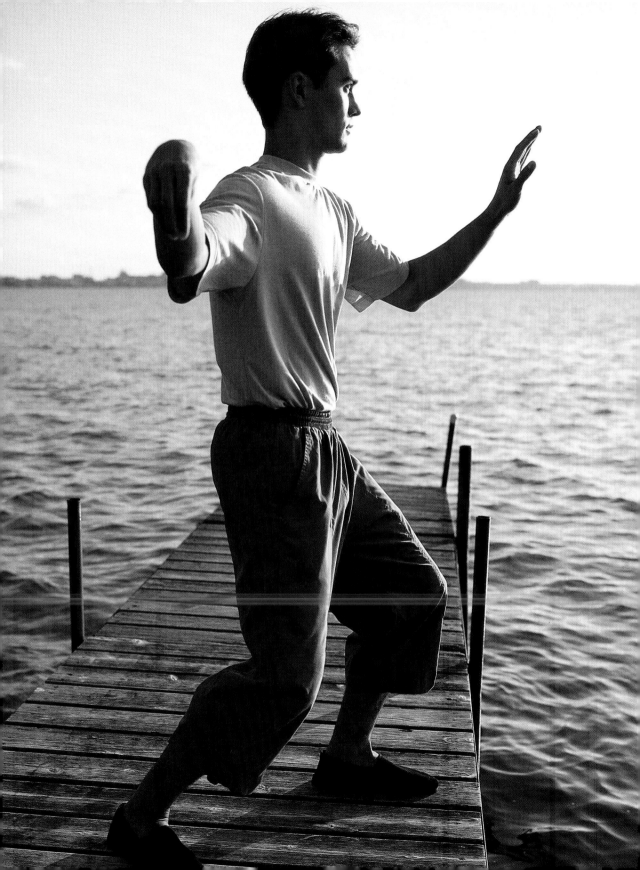

THE
FORM
PART TWO

In this part, the *Tai Chi Fold* is used in stepping back and to the side, and in changing direction. Keep your head balanced as if suspended from above as you relax and sink into your legs. Focus on staying aligned and firm as you move from your centre. Become like water flowing freely without resistance; this allows you to move both around and through obstacles lightly, without using force.

Think: fluid motion, inner tranquillity.

REPULSE MONKEY, ARMS

Move with a light and agile body. Imagine that your head is suspended from above. Your head, torso, and pelvis form a vertical column that rotates from its central axis. When this column is aligned and firmly rooted, you naturally initiate all movement from your core. Review *Basic Moves: Tai Chi Stance* (pp46–47), *Bear Roots on One Leg* (40–41), *Horse Stance* (p34), *Tai Chi Fold* (pp54–55), *Walking Skating* (p59).

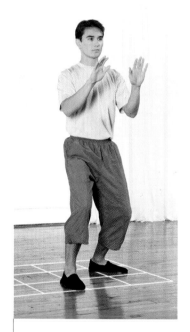

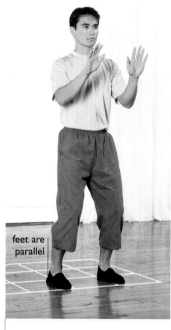

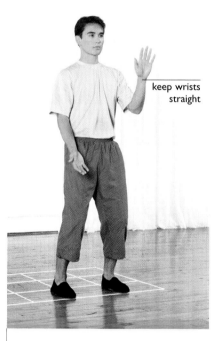

keep wrists straight

feet are parallel

1 Begin in the *Tai Chi Stance, Forward Position*, with your arms in the *Push Position*, both palms at chest height, facing forwards and slightly down.

2 Step forwards with your left foot so that both feet are parallel and hip-width apart in the *Horse Stance*. Keep your arms in the *Push Position*.

3 Lower your right arm down to your thigh with elbow slightly bent and palm facing up and forwards.

At a glance

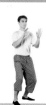 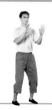 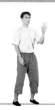 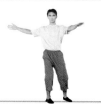 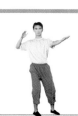

Weight forward....Step forwards...Lower arm...Fold right...Bend elbow

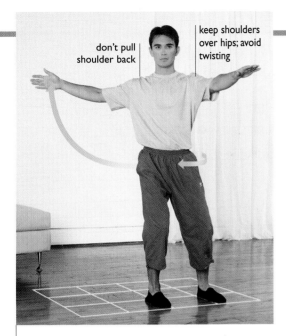

don't pull shoulder back

keep shoulders over hips; avoid twisting

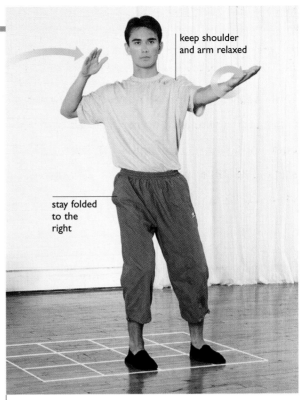

keep shoulder and arm relaxed

stay folded to the right

4 Shift your weight on to your right foot as you fold to the right by turning your pelvis and torso to the right. Simultaneously swing your right arm out to the side at shoulder height, palm facing forwards, as you extend your left arm out in front of you at shoulder height, palm facing down.

5 Bend your right elbow so that your palm faces down and your fingers point forwards. Simultaneously turn your left palm up.

6 Turn your pelvis and torso to face forwards as you shift your weight to centre so that it is evenly distributed over both feet in the *Horse Stance*. Simultaneously move your right hand down and forwards into the *Push Position*. As you do this, lower your left hand to your thigh, palm facing up and forwards. Repeat steps 4–6 on the left side so that you finish in the *Horse Stance* with your left hand in the *Push Position* and your right hand at your thigh, palm facing up and forwards. To continue, move to *Step Back to Repulse Monkey* (see over).

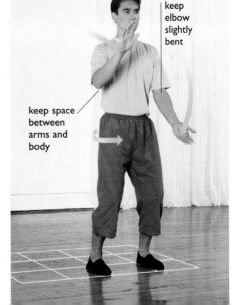

keep elbow slightly bent

keep space between arms and body

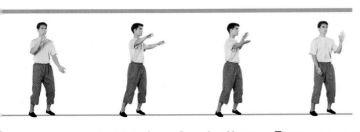

Turn centre...Fold left. ..Bend elbow...Turn centre

STEP BACK TO REPULSE MONKEY

This movement is known as "advancing while retreating". Step back from your own mind, relax, and allow your torso and pelvis to generate the circular arm movements. Review *Basic Moves: Horse Stance* (p34), *Tai Chi Fold* (54–55), *Stepping Back with the Tai Chi Fold* (pp60–61), *Walking Skating* (p59).

1 From the *Horse Stance* with left hand in the *Push Position* and right hand at your thigh, palm facing up and forwards, shift your weight entirely on to your right foot as you fold to the right by turning your pelvis and torso to the right. Simultaneously swing your right arm out to the side at shoulder height, palm facing forwards, as you extend your left arm out in front of you at shoulder height, palm facing down.

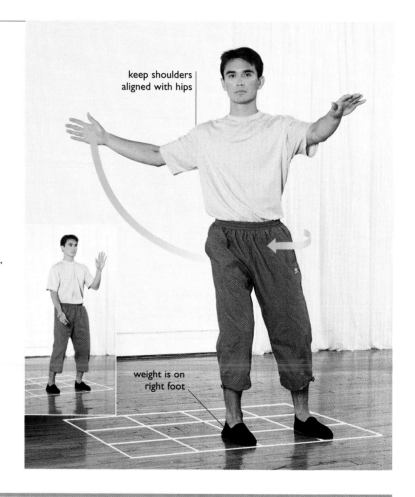

keep shoulders aligned with hips

weight is on right foot

At a glance

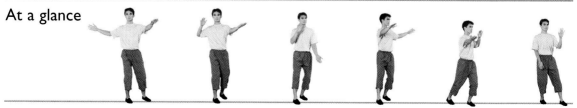

Fold right...Touch back..Shift/Turn..Fold left...Touch back..Shift/Tur

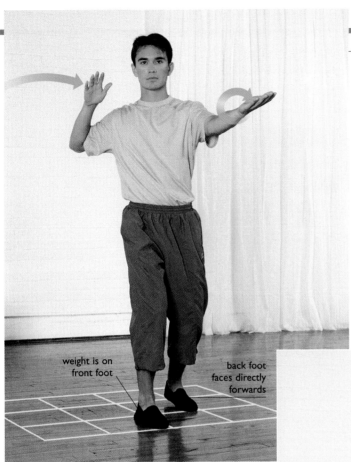

weight is on
front foot

back foot
faces directly
forwards

2 With your pelvis and torso still
folded to the right, touch back
with your left foot, slightly narrower
than shoulder-width so that your foot
is parallel to your right foot but
behind it. Simultaneously bend your
right elbow so that your palm faces
down and your fingers point forwards.
As you do this, turn your left palm up.

3 Turn your pelvis and torso to face forwards
as you shift your weight entirely on to your
left foot. Simultaneously move your right hand
down and forwards into the *Push Position.* As you
do this, lower your left hand to your thigh, palm
facing up and forwards. Repeat steps 1–3 on the
left side so that you end with your weight
entirely on your right foot with your left hand in
the *Push Position* and your right hand at your
thigh, palm facing up and forwards.
To continue, move to *Repulse Monkey to Horse
Stance* (see over).

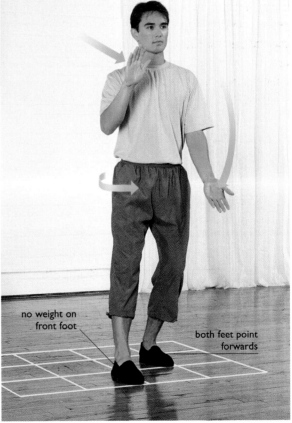

no weight on
front foot

both feet point
forwards

REPULSE MONKEY TO HORSE STANCE

Relax your lower back to make your legs more powerful and your whole body more stable. In the martial arts application of this move, one arm pushes as the other strikes down. Review *Basic Moves: Stepping Back with the Tai Chi Fold* (pp60–61), *Walking Skating* (p59), *Horse Stance* (p34).

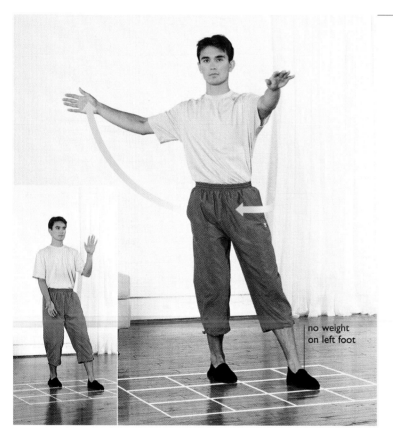

no weight
on left foot

1 With your weight entirely on your right foot, your left hand in the *Push Position* and your right hand at your thigh, palm facing up and forwards, fold to the right by turning your pelvis and torso to the right. Simultaneously swing your right arm out to the side at shoulder height with palm facing forwards, as you extend your left arm forwards at shoulder height, palm facing down.

At a glance

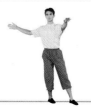 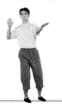 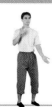

Fold right.............Step parallel.........Shift/Turn

2 Move your left foot back so that both feet are parallel and hip-width apart in the *Horse Stance* with the *Tai Chi Fold*. Keep your weight entirely on your right foot with your pelvis and torso facing to the right. Simultaneously bend your right elbow so that your palm faces down and your fingers point forwards as you turn your left palm up.

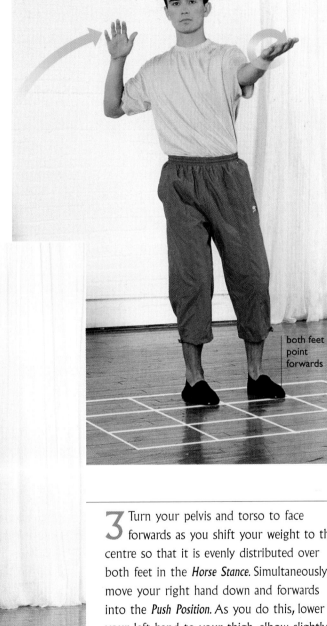

both feet point forwards

ep wrists
laxed and
aight

3 Turn your pelvis and torso to face forwards as you shift your weight to the centre so that it is evenly distributed over both feet in the *Horse Stance*. Simultaneously move your right hand down and forwards into the *Push Position*. As you do this, lower your left hand to your thigh, elbow slightly bent, palm facing up and forwards.
To continue, move to *Cloud Hands, Arms* (see over).

CLOUD HANDS, ARMS

Remain relaxed and rooted to the earth as your body moves like a floating cloud. Imagine that you are holding a cloud between your hands. Close your eyes and move your hands to face your belly and chest. Then open your eyes to see whether you have sensed the position accurately. Review *Basic Moves: Tai Chi Fold* (pp54–55), *Moving the Moon* (pp56–57).

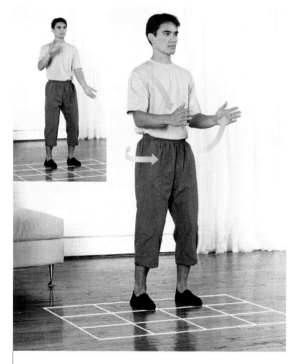

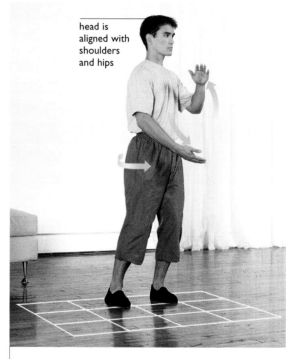

head is aligned with shoulders and hips

1 From the *Horse Stance* with your right arm in the *Push Position* and your left hand at your thigh, begin turning your pelvis and torso to the left as you shift more of your weight on to your left foot. Simultaneously move your hands so that your palms face each other in front of you.

2 Fold to the left, turning your pelvis and torso to the left diagonal as you shift your weight entirely on to your left foot. Simultaneously move your left hand to chest height, palm facing down, and your right hand to belly height, palm facing up, as if holding a large ball.

At a glance

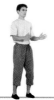 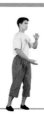 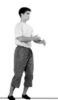 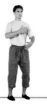 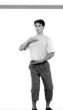

Move arms...Shift/Fold.........Move arms.....Turn centre...Shift/Fol

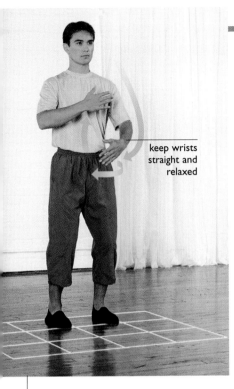

keep wrists straight and relaxed

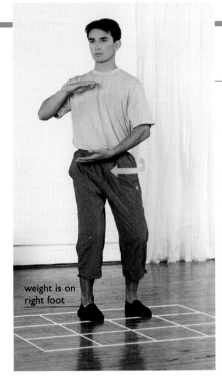

weight is on right foot

4 Shift your weight entirely on to your right foot as you fold to the right by turning your pelvis and torso to to the right. Simultaneously move your hands to face each other with your right hand at chest height, palm facing down, and your left hand at belly height, palm facing up.

3 Raise your right hand on the inside as you lower your left hand on the outside. Then turn your pelvis and torso to face forwards as you shift your weight evenly over both feet in the *Horse Stance*. Simultaneously turn your right hand so that your palm faces your chest and your left hand so that your palm faces your belly in the *Cloud Hands Position*.

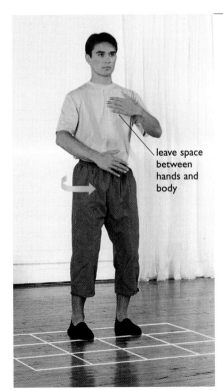

leave space between hands and body

5 Raise your left hand on the inside as you lower your right hand on the outside. Then turn your pelvis and torso to face forwards as you shift your weight evenly over both feet in the *Horse Stance*. Simultaneously turn your left hand so that your palm faces your chest and your right hand so your palm faces your belly in the *Cloud Hands Position*. To continue, move to *Cloud Hands* (see over).

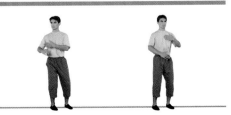

...Move arms.........Turn centre

CLOUD HANDS

Sink your weight entirely on to your stable leg, and let the other be completely weightless, or "empty". This is called separating yin and yang. When you separate your weight, you can turn lightly without using force. Remain balanced and well rooted. Keep your wrists straight and your hands relaxed. Review *Basic Moves: Tai Chi Fold* (pp54–55), *Moving the Moon* (pp56–57), *Stepping Sideways with the Tai Chi Fold* (pp62–63).

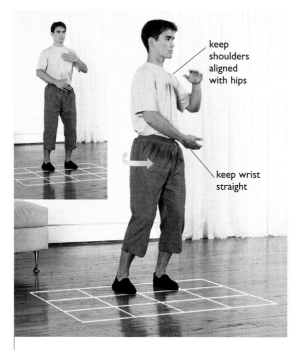

keep shoulders aligned with hips

keep wrist straight

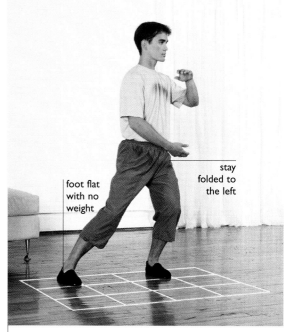

foot flat with no weight

stay folded to the left

1 From the *Horse Stance* with arms in the *Cloud Hands Position*, fold to the left by turning your pelvis and torso as you shift your weight entirely on to your left foot. Simultaneously turn your arms to face each other as if holding a large ball.

2 Keeping your weight entirely on your left foot, step to the right, wider than hip width, with your right foot. Both feet are parallel and point forwards. Your arms remain in the same position.

At a glance

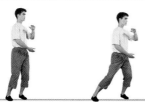
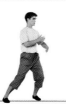
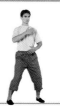
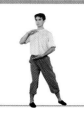

Fold left.........Step out........Move arms......Shift centre......Fold right...

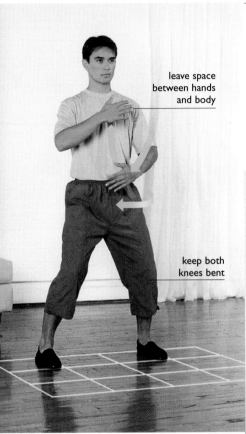

leave space
between hands
and body

keep both
knees bent

3 Raise your right hand on the inside as you lower your left hand on the outside. Then turn your pelvis and torso to face forwards as you shift your weight to centre so that it is evenly distributed over both feet in the *Horse Stance*. Simultaneously move your hands so that your right palm faces your chest and your left palm faces your belly in the *Cloud Hands Position*.

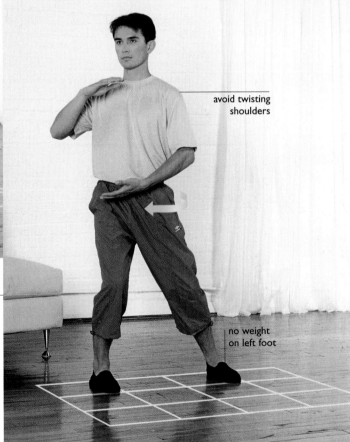

avoid twisting
shoulders

no weight
on left foot

4 Fold to the right by turning your pelvis and torso to the right as you shift your weight entirely on to your right foot. Simultaneously turn your hands to face each other as if holding a large ball.

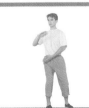 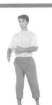 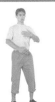 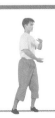

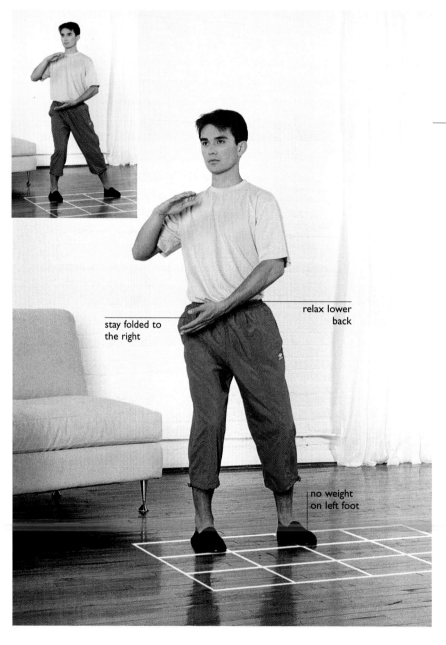

stay folded to
the right

relax lower
back

no weight
on left foot

5 Keeping all your weight on your right foot, step in with your left foot so that your feet are hip-width apart, parallel, and pointing forwards. Keep your arms in the same position.

At a glance

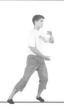 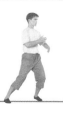 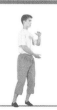 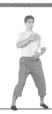

..Fold left.........Step out..........Move arms.............Shift centre.......

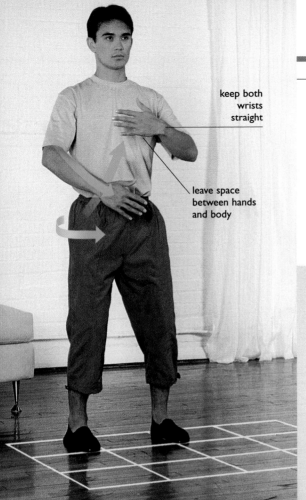

keep both wrists straight

leave space between hands and body

6 Raise your left hand on the inside as you lower your right hand on the outside. Then shift your weight so that it is evenly distributed over both feet as you turn your pelvis and torso to face forwards in the *Horse Stance*. Simultaneously move your hands so that your left palm faces your chest and your right palm faces your belly in the *Cloud Hands Position*.

keep both wrists straight

no weight on right foot

7 Fold to the left by turning your pelvis and torso to the left as you shift your weight entirely on to your left foot. Simultaneously move your hands to face each other with your left hand at chest height, palm facing down, and your right hand at belly height, palm facing up. To continue, move to *Single Whip* (see over).

 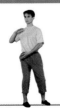 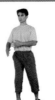 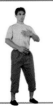 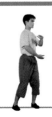

....Fold right..........Step in............Move arms.........Shift centre.......Fold left

SINGLE WHIP

Move slowly and deliberately in a flowing sequence. Your torso rotates like a wheel, directing the action into the arms, hands, and fingers. In the martial art application of the *Single Whip*, the wrist of the *Crane Beak Hand* is actually used to strike. Review *Basic Moves: Horse Stance to Tai Chi Stance* (pp64–65).

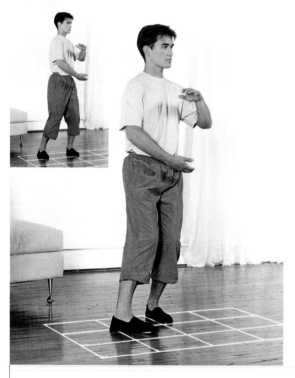

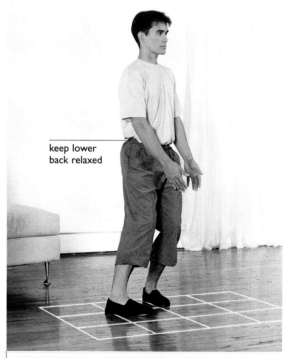

keep lower
back relaxed

1 From the *Horse Stance with Tai Chi Fold*, your hands facing each other in front of you as if holding a large ball, step forwards with your right foot pointing diagonally inwards.

2 Lower your left hand so that both hands face each other at your left hip.

At a glance

Step forwards.......Lower hand.......Shift right......Fold right......Turn centre..

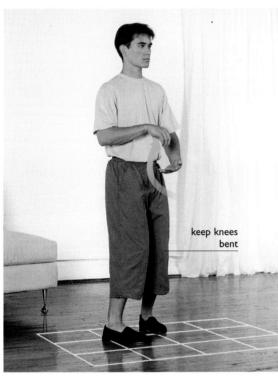

keep knees
bent

3 Begin shifting your
weight on to your right
foot as you raise your
hands to belly height, left
palm up, right hand fingers
pointing down.

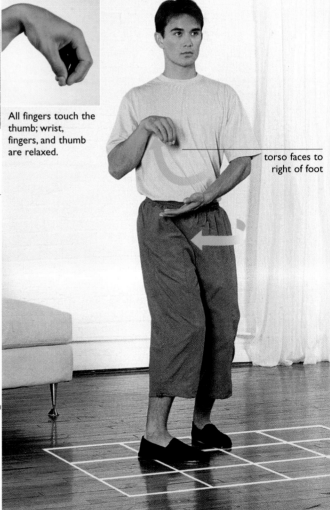

All fingers touch the
thumb; wrist,
fingers, and thumb
are relaxed.

torso faces to
right of foot

4 Fold to the right by turning your pelvis
and torso to the right as you shift your
weight entirely on to your right foot. As you
do this, move your right hand to chest height
with elbow slightly bent, wrist down, and fingers
touching your thumb in the *Crane Beak Hand*.
Simultaneously move your left hand to belly
height, palm facing up.

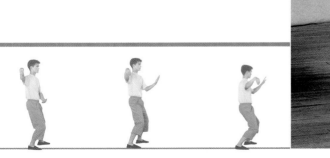

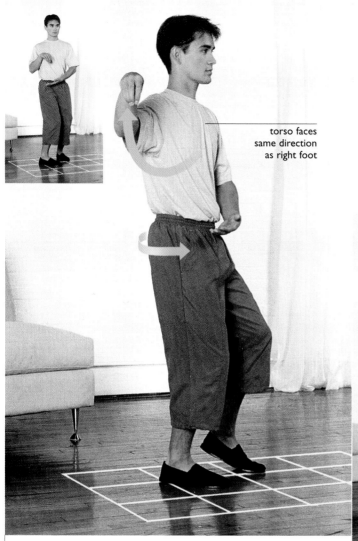

torso faces
same direction
as right foot

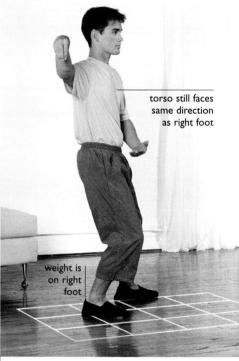

torso still faces
same direction
as right foot

weight is
on right
foot

5 Turn your pelvis and torso to face the direction of your right foot as you pivot on the ball of your left foot. Simultaneously extend your right *Crane Beak Hand* out to your side at shoulder height.

6 Step forwards on to your left foot and hip-distance from your right heel in the *Tai Chi Stance, Back Position.* Keep your arms in the same position.

At a glance

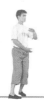 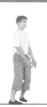 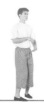 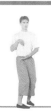

Step forwards..........Lower hand........Shift right...............Fold right....

7 Begin shifting your weight on to your left foot as you raise your left arm in front of you, palm facing you. Keep your right arm in the same position.

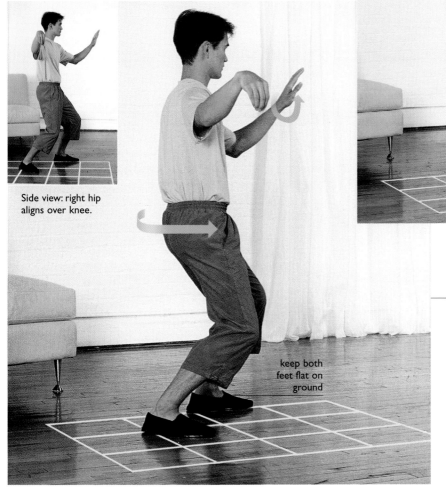

keep elbow low

Side view: right hip aligns over knee.

keep both feet flat on ground

8 Shift 70 percent of your weight on to your left foot as you turn your pelvis and torso to face forwards in the *Tai Chi Stance, Forward Position*. Simultaneously turn your left palm to face forwards and slightly down in the *Push Position*. Your right hand remains in the *Crane Beak Position* extended at your right side. Finish here, or proceed to *Snake Slides Down* (see pp120–121).

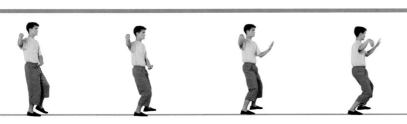

......Turn centre.......Step left.........Shift left.........Shift/Turn

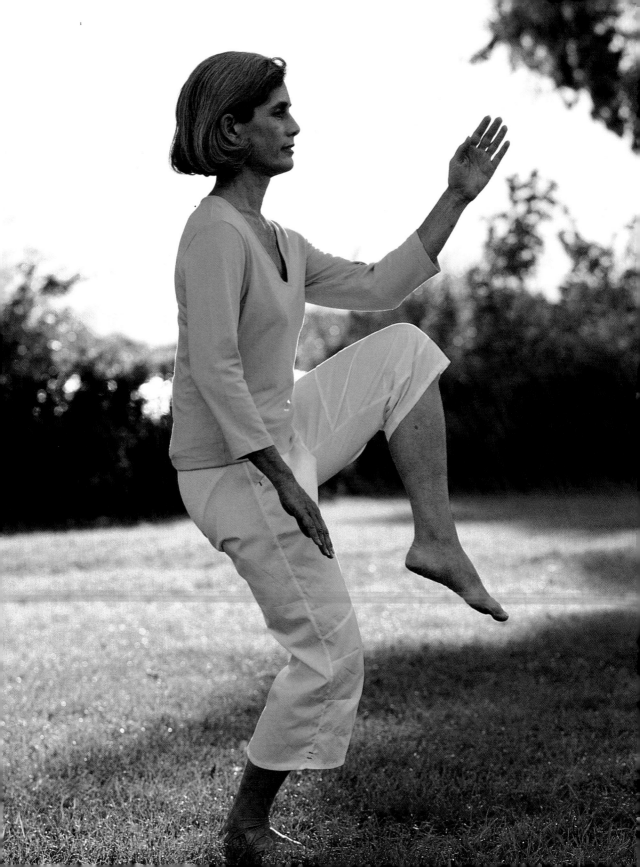

THE
FORM

PART THREE

In this final part you practise power moves in the tai chi stance and more advanced postures that require strength, flexibility, and good balance. Remain relaxed and yet rooted to the earth. Balance your head, torso, and pelvis as if they float on your legs. Let your body become as strong as an oak and as flexible as a willow. Let your mind become as clear as still water. This is the essence of tai chi.

SNAKE SLIDES DOWN

Keep your mind quiet and focused. Here, you use the *Tai Chi Fold* to withdraw your left arm and then the *Forward Transition* to strike forwards. Review *Basic Moves: Tai Chi Stance with Fold* (pp76–77), *Tai Chi Stance, Forward Transition* (pp50–51).

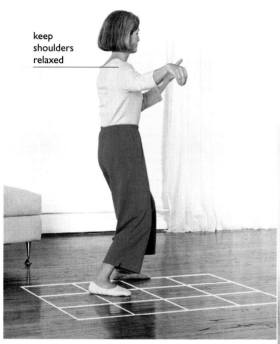

keep shoulders relaxed

1 Begin in the *Tai Chi Stance, Forward Position* with your left hand in the *Push Position*. Your right arm is extended to your right at shoulder height with your hand in the *Crane Beak Position*.

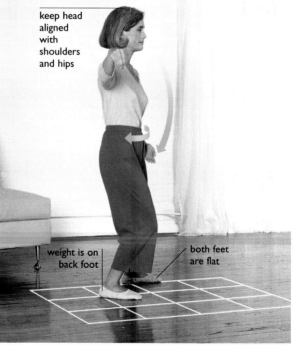

keep head aligned with shoulders and hips

weight is on back foot

both feet are flat

2 Turn your pelvis and torso to the right as you shift your weight entirely on to your right foot to move into the *Tai Chi Stance with Fold*. Simultaneously move your left hand to the inside of your left thigh, palm facing right. Your right arm remains in the same position.

At a glance

   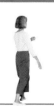

Weight forward........Shift/Turn...........Turn left........Shift forwards

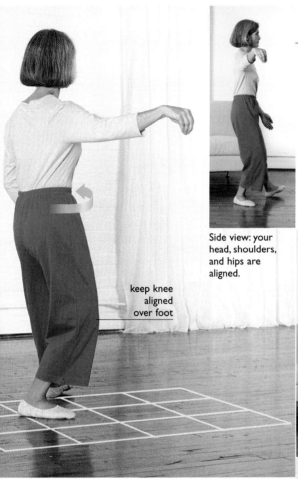

keep knee
aligned
over foot

Side view: your
head, shoulders,
and hips are
aligned.

3 Turn your pelvis and torso to
your left as you pivot on your
left heel so that your left foot points
diagonally to the left. Keep both arms
in the same position.

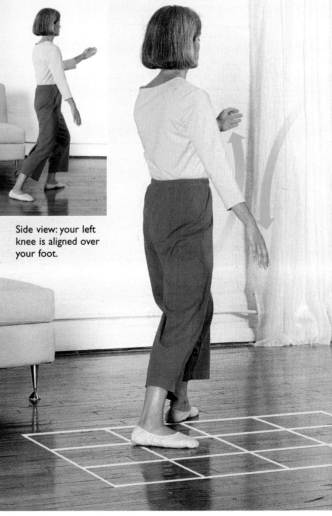

Side view: your left
knee is aligned over
your foot.

4 Shift your weight on to your
left foot to move into the
Forward Transition. Simultaneously
swing your left arm forwards as
you lower your right arm to your
side and open your hand.
To continue, move to *Golden
Pheasant Stands on One Leg* (see over).

GOLDEN PHEASANT STANDS ON ONE LEG

Here your knee and fingers strike simultaneously – to help your balance, feel into the sole of your foot, and relax your lower back so that your tailbone feels heavy. To be both stable and full of energy, feel uplifted at your crown. Review *Basic Moves: High Step* (pp67–68).

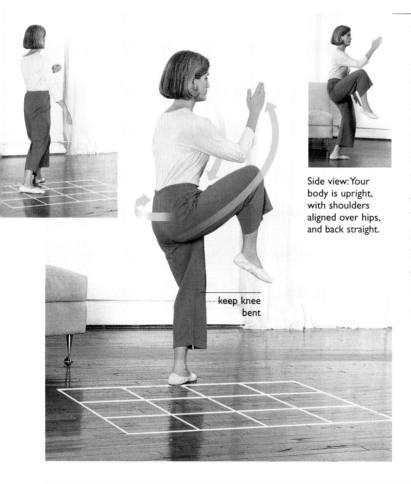

keep knee bent

Side view: Your body is upright, with shoulders aligned over hips, and back straight.

1 From the *Forward Transition*, shift your weight entirely on to your left foot. Raise your right knee directly in front of you in the *High Step Position* as you turn your pelvis and torso to face forwards. If you have trouble balancing, lower your right leg so that your toes touch the ground to steady you. Simultaneously bend your right elbow and move your hand to neck level with fingers at midline pointing up, palm facing left. As you do this, lower your left arm so that your hand faces down and forwards, parallel to your left thigh. Your arms are in the *Golden Pheasant Position.*

At a glance

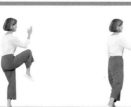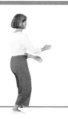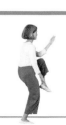

Raise knee.........Touch back......Shift back..........Raise knee

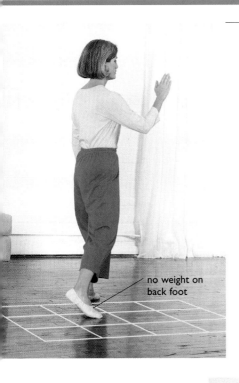

no weight on
back foot

2 Touch back diagonally with your right foot. Your arms remain in the same position.

3 Shift your weight entirely on to your back, right foot. Simultaneously begin lowering your right arm and raising your left arm.

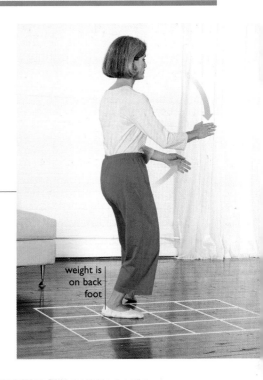

weight is
on back
foot

4 Keeping your weight entirely on your right foot, raise your left knee directly in front of you in the *High Step Position*. Simultaneously bend your left elbow and move your hand to neck level with fingers at midline pointing up, palm facing right. As you do this, lower your right arm so that your hand faces down and forwards, parallel to your right thigh in the *Golden Pheasant Position*.
To continue, move to *Separate Arms and Kick* (see over).

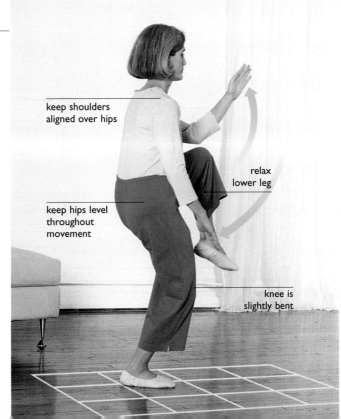

keep shoulders
aligned over hips

keep hips level
throughout
movement

relax
lower leg

knee is
slightly bent

SEPARATE ARMS AND KICK

To keep your movements both relaxed and lively, imagine that your bones are loosely strung together like a string of pearls. This stimulates the flow of qi within your body. Visualize stretching a rubber band or a beam of light between your hands as you move them apart. Review *Basic Moves: Toe Kick* (pp72–73), *Dancing Crane* (pp74–75).

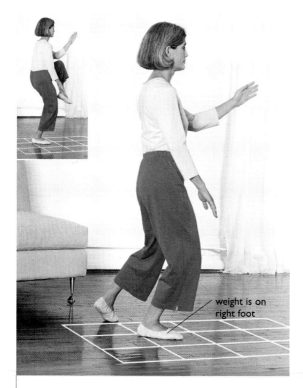

weight is on right foot

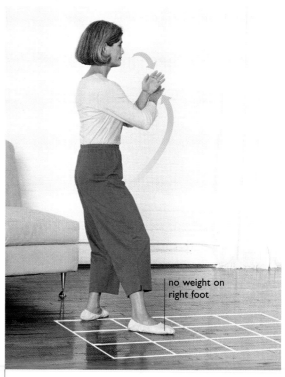

no weight on right foot

1 From the *High Step Position*, arms in the *Golden Pheasant Position*, touch back diagonally with your left foot, toes first. As you do this, begin lowering your left arm, keeping your right arm in the same position.

2 Shift your weight entirely on to your left foot. Simultaneously move your arms so that your wrists cross at chest height with your right arm on the outside and your left arm on the inside. Your palms face to the sides and down.

At a glance

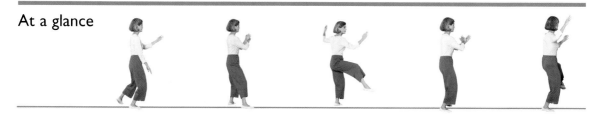

Touch back..........Shift back...........Kick.........Shift right.........Kick

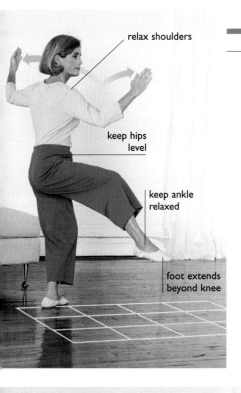

relax shoulders

keep hips level

keep ankle relaxed

foot extends beyond knee

3 Look to the right as you raise your right leg to the right diagonal in the *Toe Kick Position*. Simultaneously move your right arm over your right thigh so that your elbow is at chest height, and extend you left arm to the side of your body with your elbow at shoulder height. The palms of your hands face each other in the *Separate Arms Position*.

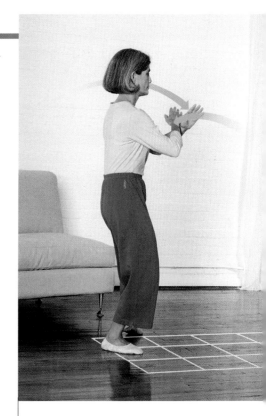

4 Keeping your weight entirely on your left foot, touch back with your right foot. Then shift your weight entirely on to your right foot. Simultaneously move your arms so that your wrists cross at chest height with your left arm on the outside and your right arm on the inside. Your palms face to the sides and down.

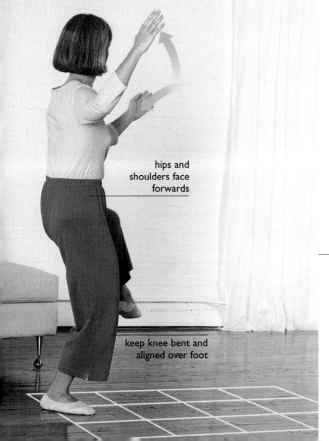

hips and shoulders face forwards

keep knee bent and aligned over foot

5 Look to the left as you raise your left leg to the left diagonal in the *Toe Kick Position*. Simultaneously move your left arm over your left thigh so that your elbow is at chest height, and extend your right arm to the side of your body with your elbow at shoulder height. Your hands face each other in the *Separate Arms Position*.
To continue, move to *Brush Knee (Left)* (see over).

BRUSH KNEE (LEFT)

Tai chi uses mind, not force. Keep your arms both relaxed and full of energy, blocking with your left hand and pushing with your right. Move with minimal effort; your hands are a conduit for the action. Review *Basic Moves: Tai Chi Stance* (pp46–47), *Tai Chi Stance with Fold* (pp76–77).

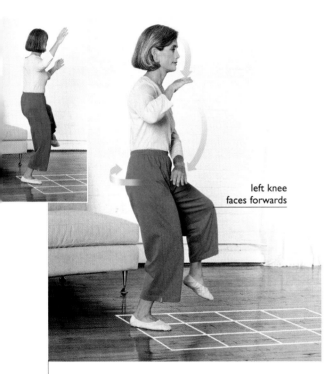

left knee faces forwards

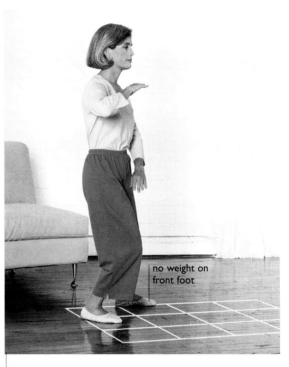

no weight on front foot

1 From the *Toe Kick Position* with arms in the *Separate Arms Position*, turn your pelvis and torso to the right. Simultaneously bend your right elbow so that your fingers point forwards and circle your left hand to your right hip, palm facing down.

2 Place your left foot hip-distance from your right heel in the *Tai Chi Stance, Back Position*. Simultaneously lower your left hand down in front of your right thigh with palm facing left.

At a glance

Turn right.......Step left.........Align knee.....Shift/Turn..........Fold righ

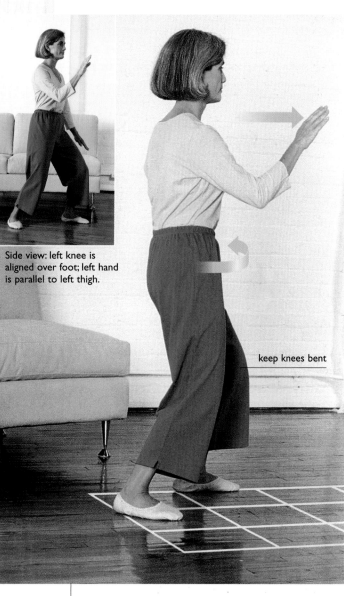

left knee aligns over centre of foot

Side view: left knee is aligned over foot; left hand is parallel to left thigh.

keep knees bent

3 Bend your left knee slightly so that it is directly over the centre of your foot. Your arms remain in the same position.

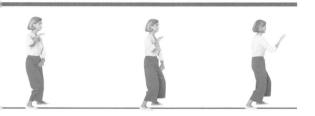

4 Turn your pelvis and torso to face the direction of your left foot as you shift 70 percent of your weight forwards to move into the *Tai Chi Stance, Forward Position*. Simultaneously move your arms into the *Brush Knee Position* by moving your right hand forwards into the *Push Position*, as you move your left hand parallel to your left thigh, palm down, fingers facing down and forwards.

Move arms.......Align knee......Shift/Turn

5 Fold to the right by turning your pelvis and torso to the right as you shift your weight entirely on to your right foot to move into the *Tai Chi Stance with Fold*. Simultaneously swing your right arm down and out to your side at shoulder height, palm facing forwards, as you circle your left hand to the front of your right hip, palm facing down.

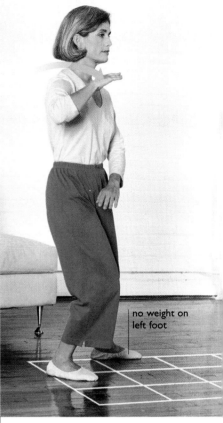

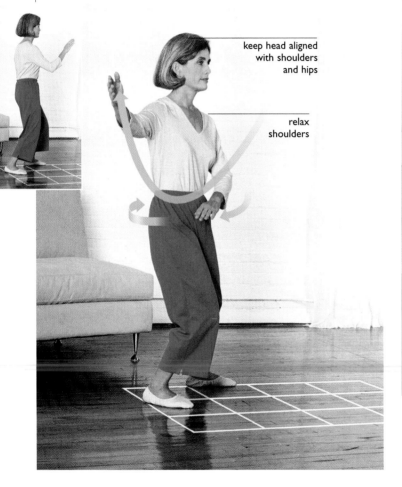

keep head aligned
with shoulders
and hips

relax
shoulders

no weight on
left foot

6 Bend your right elbow to move your hand so that your fingers point in the same direction as your left foot. Simultaneously move your left hand down in front of your right thigh, palm facing left.

At a glance

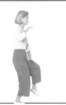
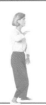

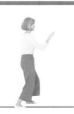
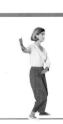

Turn right........Step left.........Align knee......Shift/Turn........Fold right.

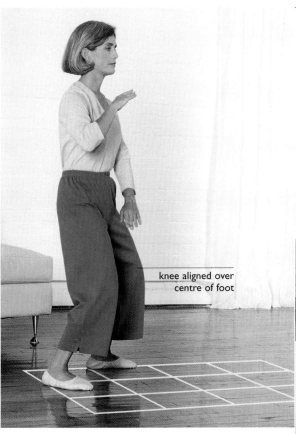

knee aligned over
centre of foot

7 Bend your left knee slightly so that it is directly over the centre of your foot. Your arms remain in the same position.

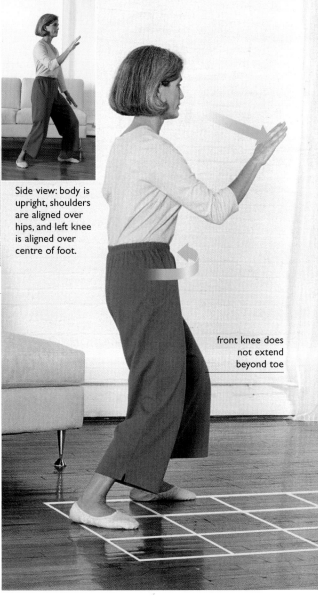

Side view: body is upright, shoulders are aligned over hips, and left knee is aligned over centre of foot.

front knee does not extend beyond toe

8 Turn your pelvis and torso to face the direction of your left foot as you shift 70 percent of your weight forwards to move into the *Tai Chi Stance, Forward Position*. Simultaneously, move your arms into the *Brush Knee Position* by moving your right hand forwards into the *Push Position*, as you move your left hand parallel to your left thigh, palm down, fingers facing down and forwards.

To continue, move to *Brush Knee (Right)* (see over).

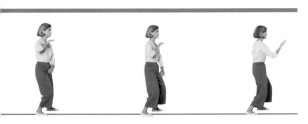

....Move arms.....Align knee.....Shift/Turn

BRUSH KNEE (RIGHT)

After the forward transition, *Brush Knee* is now repeated with the right foot forward. Relax your arms; feel how the movement is motivated by the turning of your torso. Review *Basic Moves: Tai Chi Stance, Forward Transition* (pp50–51), *Tai Chi Stance with Fold* (pp76–77).

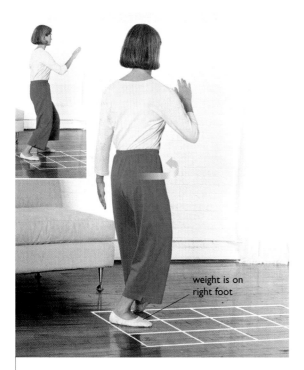

weight is on right foot

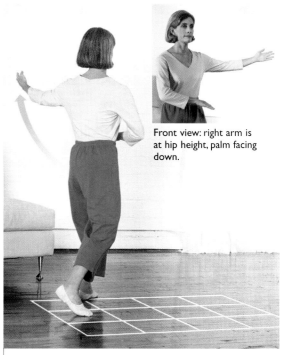

Front view: right arm is at hip height, palm facing down.

1 From the *Tai Chi Stance, Forward Position*, with arms in the *Brush Knee Position*, shift your weight entirely on to your right foot as you turn your pelvis, torso, and left foot to the left diagonal, pivoting on your left heel. Simultaneously turn your left palm to face forwards and your right palm to face left and slightly down.

2 Shift your weight on to your left foot to move into the *Forward Transition*. Simultaneously swing your left arm out to your side at shoulder height, palm facing forwards, as you move your right arm in front of your left hip, palm facing down.

At a glance

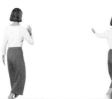

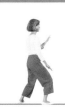

Shift/Turn.......Shift forwards.....Step forwards....Align knee.......Shift/Tur

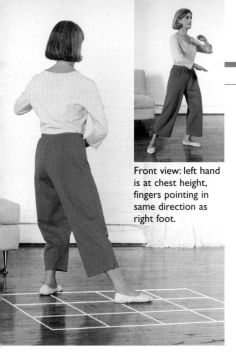

Front view: left hand is at chest height, fingers pointing in same direction as right foot.

3 Step forwards with your right foot into the *Tai Chi Stance, Back Position*. Simultaneously bend your left elbow so that your fingers point forwards as you move your right hand down in front of your left thigh, palm facing down.

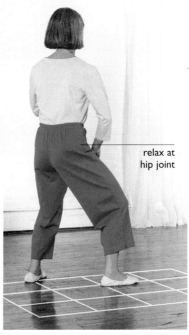

relax at hip joint

4 Bend your right knee slightly so that it is directly over the centre of your foot. Your arms remain in the same position.

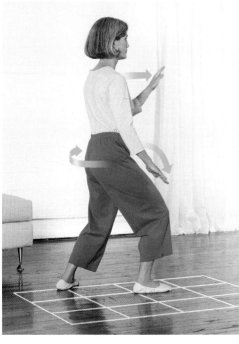

5 Turn your pelvis and torso to face the direction of your right foot as you shift 70 percent of your weight on to your right foot to move into the *Tai Chi Stance, Forward Position*. Simultaneously move your arms into the *Brush Knee Position* by moving your left hand forwards into the *Push Position*, palm facing forwards and slightly down, as you move your right hand parallel to your right thigh, fingers facing down and forwards.

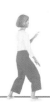

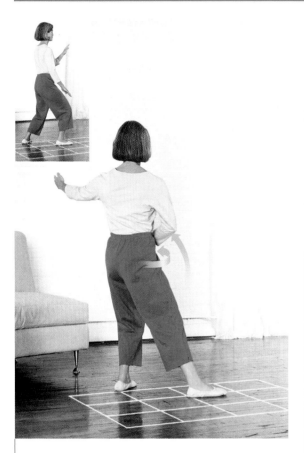

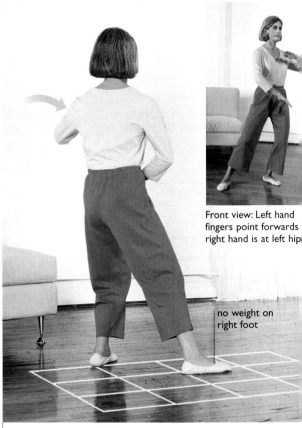

Front view: Left hand
fingers point forwards
right hand is at left hip

no weight on
right foot

6 From the *Tai Chi Stance, Forward Position*, with
arms in the *Brush Knee Position*, fold to the left
by rotating your pelvis and torso to the left as
you shift your weight entirely on to your left
foot to move into the *Tai Chi Stance with the Fold*.
Simultaneously swing your left arm out to your
side at shoulder height, palm facing forwards, as
you circle your right hand to your left hip,
palm facing down.

7 Stay folded to the left with your weight entirely
on your left foot. Bend your left elbow so that
your fingers point forwards in the same direction
as your right foot as you move your right hand
down in front of your left thigh, palm facing right.

At a glance

Shift/Turn.......Shift forwards......Step forwards.....Align knee......Shift/Tur▸

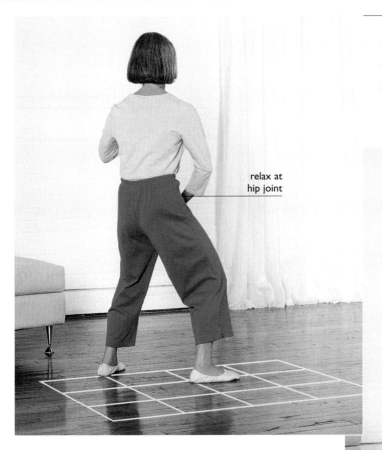

relax at
hip joint

8 Bend your right knee so that it aligns directly over the centre of your foot. Your arms remain in the same position.

9 Turn your pelvis and torso to face the direction of your right foot as you shift 70 percent of your weight on to your right foot to move into the *Tai Chi Stance, Forward Position.* Simultaneously move your arms into the *Brush Knee Position* by moving your left hand forwards into the *Push Position,* palm facing forwards and slightly down, as you move your right hand parallel to your right thigh, fingers facing down and forwards.
To continue, move to *Punch* (see over).

PUNCH

Here you block with your left arm, then punch with your right fist. Be both still and alert, like a cat watching a mouse. To act effectively, relax the mind and the body. Review *Basic Moves: Tai Chi Stance, Forward Transition* (pp50–51), *Tai Chi Stance* (pp46–47).

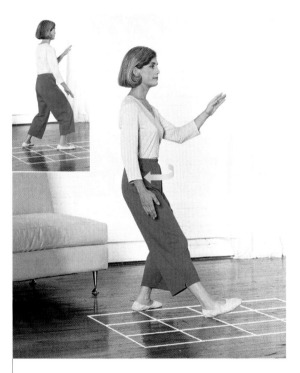

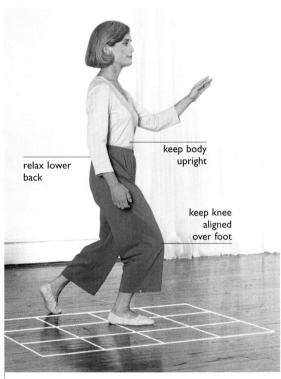

relax lower
back

keep body
upright

keep knee
aligned
over foot

1 From the *Tai Chi Stance, Forward Position*, arms in the *Brush Knee Position*, shift your weight entirely on to your left foot as you turn your pelvis, torso, and right foot to the right diagonal, pivoting on your right heel. Simultaneously turn your right palm to face forwards and your left palm to face right and slightly down.

2 Shift your weight on to your right foot to move into the *Forward Transition*. Your left arm maintains the same position as you begin to curl the fingers of your right hand.

At a glance

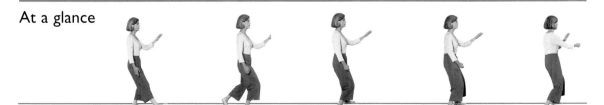

Shift/Turn.......Shift forwards...Step forwards...Align knee....Shift/Turn

3 Step forwards with your left foot into the *Tai Chi Stance, Back Position.* Simultaneously form a loose fist with your right hand. Keep your left hand in the same position.

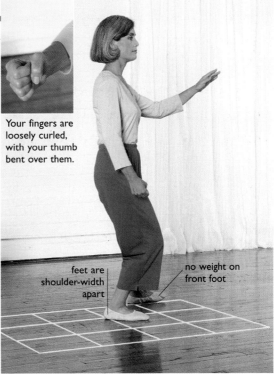

Your fingers are loosely curled, with your thumb bent over them.

feet are shoulder-width apart

no weight on front foot

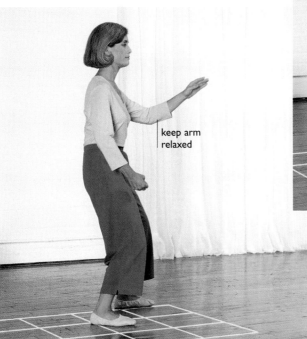

keep arm relaxed

4 Bend your left knee so that it aligns directly over the centre of your foot. Your arms remain in the same position.

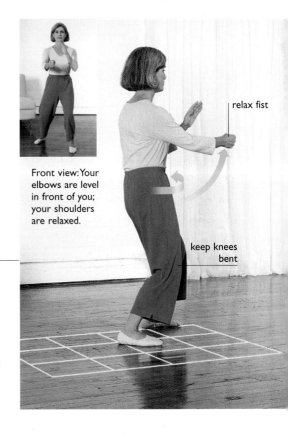

relax fist

Front view: Your elbows are level in front of you; your shoulders are relaxed.

keep knees bent

5 Turn your pelvis and torso to face the direction of your left foot as you shift 70 percent of your weight on to your left foot to move into the *Tai Chi Stance, Forward Position.* Simultaneously move your right fist forwards directly in front of you, with your forearm parallel to the ground, as you bend your left elbow so that your hand is at chest height in front of you with palm facing your right forearm. This is the *Punch Position.* To continue, move to *Withdraw and Push* (see over).

WITHDRAW AND PUSH

In this move your left hand strikes as your right hand withdraws, then both hands push. As you fold you simultaneously withdraw and wind up for the push. Review *Basic Moves: Tai Chi Stance with the Fold* (pp76–77), *Tai Chi Stance* (pp46–47).

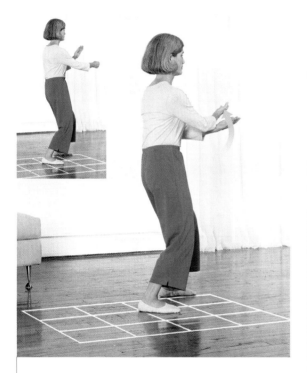

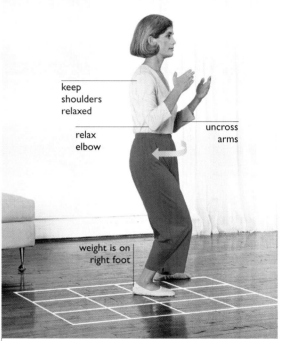

keep shoulders relaxed

relax elbow

uncross arms

weight is on right foot

1 From the *Tai Chi Stance, Forward Position*, with arms in the *Punch Position*, begin shifting your weight back on to your right foot. As you do this, cross your arms horizontally at the forearms by extending your right arm and opening your palm to face up as you lower your left hand under your right forearm, palm up.

2 Fold to the right by turning your pelvis and torso to the right diagonal as you shift your weight entirely on to your right foot in the *Tai Chi Stance with the Fold*. Simultaneously uncross your arms by drawing your right hand over your left wrist, both palms facing up and towards your body.

At a glance

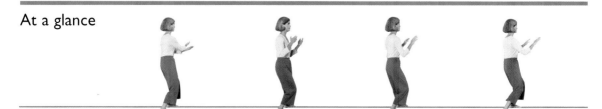

Shift back...........Fold right........Turn centre.......Shift forwards

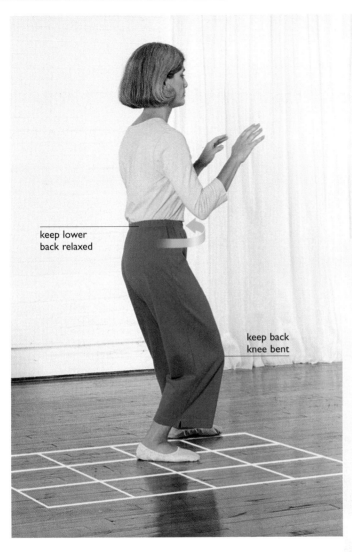

keep lower
back relaxed

keep back
knee bent

3 Turn your pelvis and torso to
face forwards in the direction of
your left foot in the *Tai Chi Stance, Back
Position*. As you do this, move your
arms into the *Push Position* by turning
both hands to face forwards with
forearms parallel to each other.

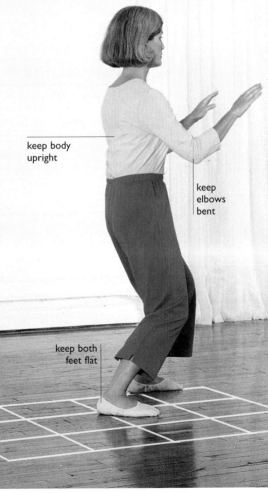

keep body
upright

keep
elbows
bent

keep both
feet flat

4 Shift 70 percent of your weight forwards on
to your left foot to move into the *Tai Chi
Stance, Forward Position*. Keep your arms in the *Push
Position*, but swing your elbows slightly forwards.
To continue, move to *Cross Hands* (see over).

CROSS HANDS

Imagine that your hands are making a rainbow as they separate, and gathering new life as they circle down and then cross in front of you. Review *Basic Moves: Tai Chi Stance to Horse Stance* (pp80–81).

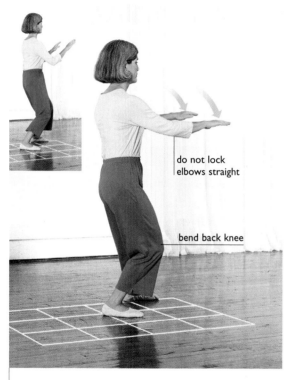

do not lock elbows straight

bend back knee

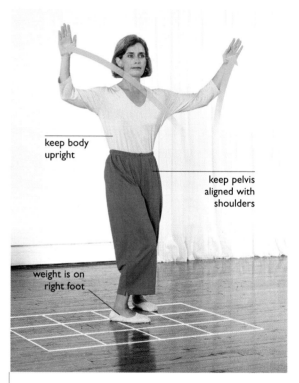

keep body upright

keep pelvis aligned with shoulders

weight is on right foot

1 From the *Tai Chi Stance, Forward Position*, with arms in the *Push Position*, shift your weight entirely on to your right foot to move into the *Tai Chi Stance, Back Position*. As you do this, straighten your elbows so that both palms face down and your fingers point forwards.

2 Keeping your weight entirely on your right foot, fold to the right by turning your pelvis, torso, and left foot 90° to the right, pivoting on your left heel. Simultaneously raise your arms to head level at your sides with fingers pointing up and out and palms facing forwards.

At a glance

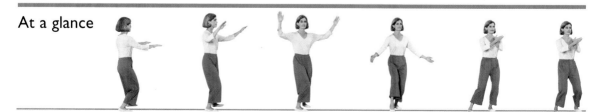

Shift right................Fold right...........Shift left...Step back....Shift centr

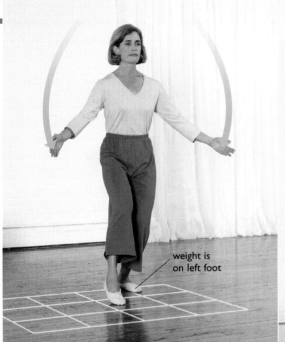

weight is
on left foot

3 Shift your weight entirely on to your left
foot as you pivot on the toes of your
right foot to face the same direction as your
left foot. Simultaneously circle both arms down
in front of you so that your fingers point down
and out and your palms face forwards.

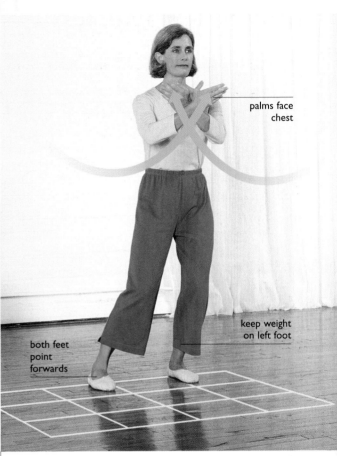

palms face
chest

both feet
point
forwards

keep weight
on left foot

4 Step back with your right foot so that it is
parallel to and hip-distance from your left foot.
As you do this, move your right arm under your left
as you bend your elbows and turn your palms to face
your chest, fingers pointing up and to the diagonal.
Your arms are in the *Cross Hands Position.*

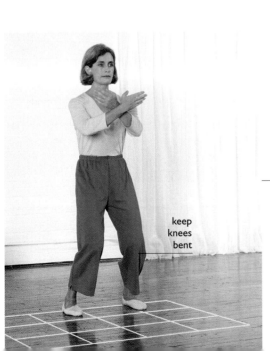

keep
knees
bent

5 Move to the *Horse Stance* by shifting
your weight to the centre so that it
is evenly distributed over both feet with
knees bent. Your arms remain in the *Cross
Hands Position.*
To continue, move to *Closing Move* (see over).

CLOSING MOVE

Your arms return to your sides as you bring the Form to a close. Focus on breathing slowly and deeply. Consider the unity of all things. Finally, be still and at peace as you return to your starting point. Review *Basic Moves: Horse Stance* (p34), *Stable and Open* (pp42–43).

1 From the *Horse Stance* with arms in the *Cross Hands Position*, straighten your knees slightly. Simultaneously lower both arms so that they hang relaxed at your sides with your elbows slightly bent, wrists straight, and fingers facing down and slightly forwards in the *Wu Chi Position*. Pause and breathe.

2 Bend your knees, and shift your weight entirely on to your left foot. Simultaneously turn your pelvis and torso to the right diagonal, pivoting on your right heel so that your foot points diagonally outward in the *Stable and Open Position*. Simultaneously turn your palms to face each other.

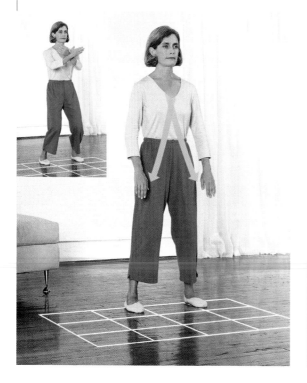

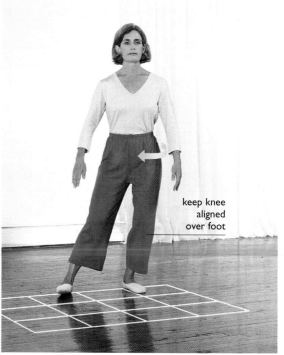

keep knee
aligned
over foot

At a glance

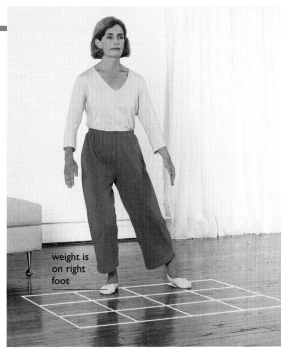

weight is
on right
foot

3 Shift your weight entirely on to
your right foot. Keep your arms
in the same position.

4 Move your left foot into diagonal position
next to your right foot so that your heels
are together in a "V" position. Your arms
maintain the same position.

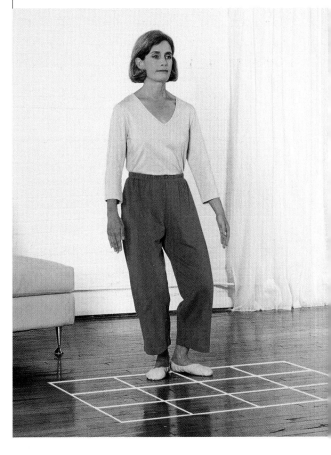

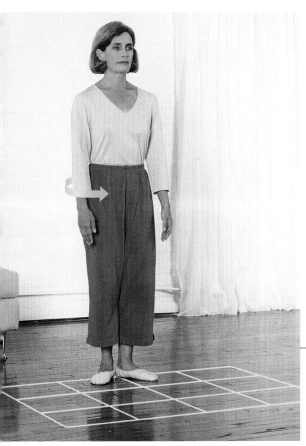

5 Shift your weight to the centre as you turn
your pelvis and torso to face forwards, then
straighten your knees slightly. Relax your arms at
your sides, and finally, take a moment to focus on
your breathing.

THE FORM SUMMARY

This summary is a reference for the entire sequence of movements in the Form. Once you are familiar with these movements, refer to this summary to help remember each section, or the entire sequence of the Form. Remember to practise the warm ups (*see pp24–29*) and sensing qi (*see pp20–23*) before each session. You may want to finish with the exercises for moving and gathering qi (*see pp148–153*).

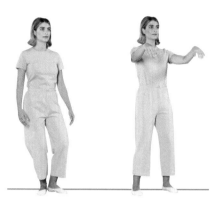

Preparation
pp88–89

Beginning
pp90–91

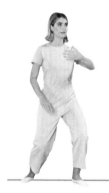

Ward off (left)
pp92–93

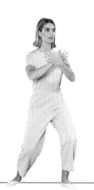

Press (left)
p94

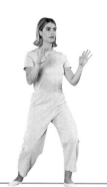

Push (left)
p95

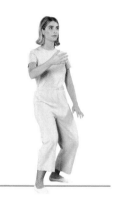

Ward off (right)
pp96–97

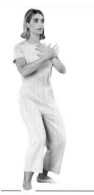

Press (right)
p98

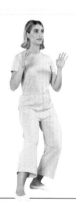

Push (right)
p99

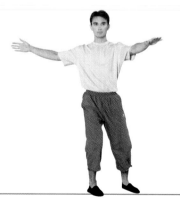

Step forward to
repulse monkey
pp102–103

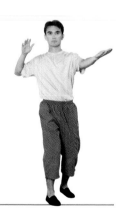

Step back to repulse
monkey
pp104–105

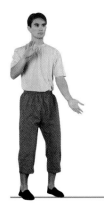
Repulse monkey to horse
stance *pp106–107*

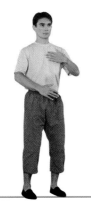
Cloud hands, arms
pp108–109

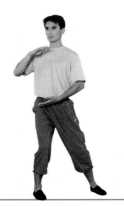
Cloud hands
pp110–113

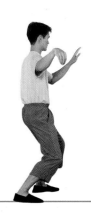
Single whip
pp114–117

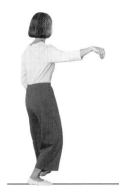
Snake slides down
pp120–121

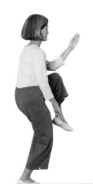
Golden pheasant
stands on one leg
pp122–123

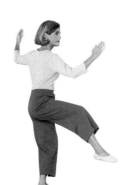
Separate arms
and kick
pp124–125

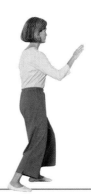
Brush knee (left)
pp126–129

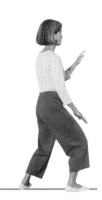
Brush knee (right)
pp130–133

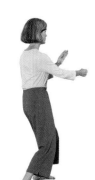
Punch
pp134–135

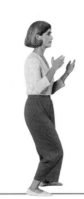
Withdraw and push
pp136–137

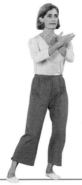
Cross hands
pp138–139

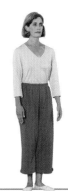
Closing move
pp140–141

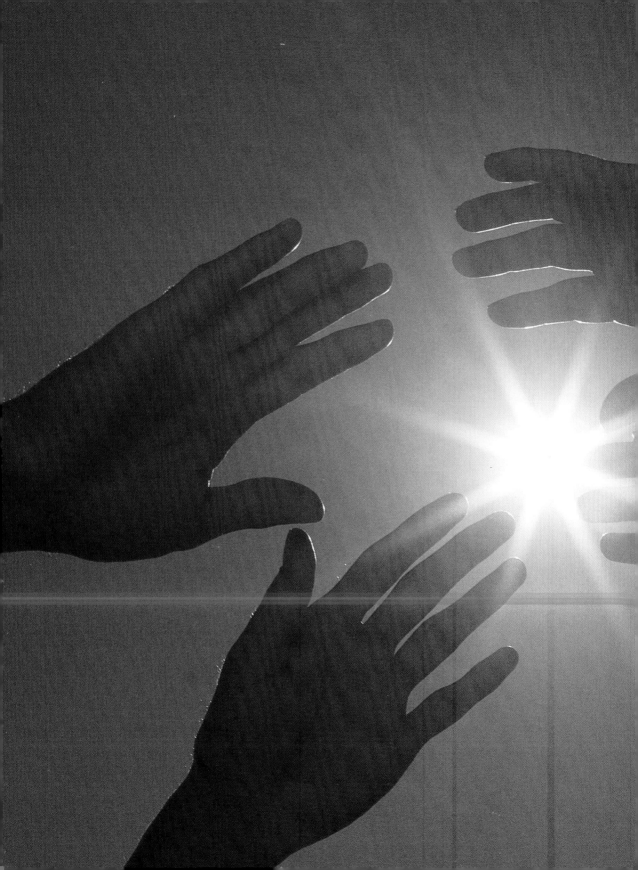

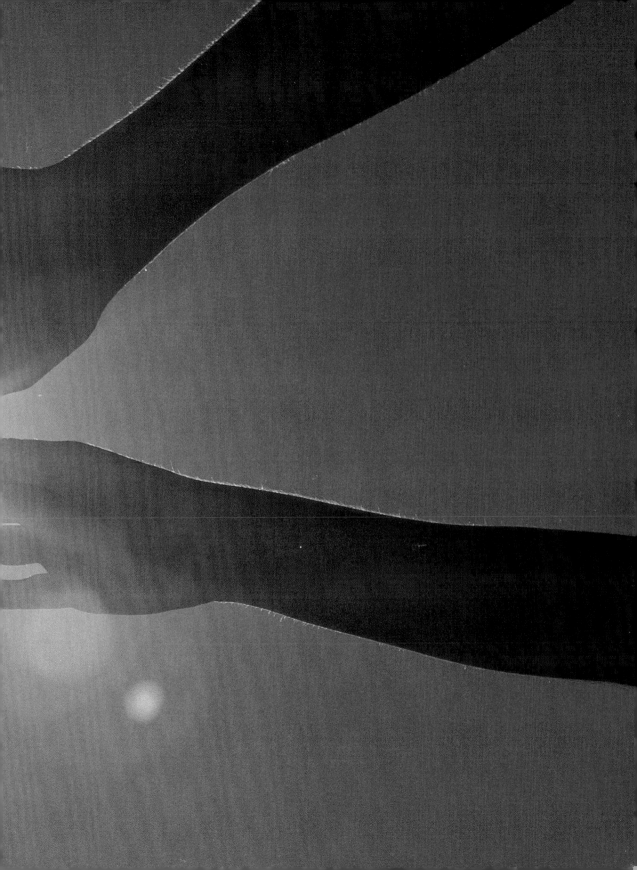

CULTIVATING QI

Qi, or "life energy", pervades the whole universe. It is the vital life force that flows through our bodies and all around us. Here you will discover how you can expand awareness of qi within your own body and more easily sense the subtle energy of the natural world and beyond. It is also useful to understand qi in terms of vital points and energy fields.

VITAL ENERGY

According to Chinese medicine, qi flows through channels, or meridians, in the body that are connected like a complex network of rivers. Along the meridians are many vital points, which correspond to the basic acupressure points used in acupuncture. There are also three reservoirs of qi or "energy fields" within the body – known as the lower, middle, and upper *dan tians* – where qi is generated and stored (*see opposite*).

The lower *dan tian* is situated deep within the belly and corresponds to the body's physical centre of gravity. It is the primary area of focus during tai chi practice. It helps you to feel connection to the earth and is responsible for feelings of personal stability, safety, and security. This is where you experience a "gut response" to something. The middle *dan tian* is situated within the chest. It is your interpersonal energy field, where you feel the pain of a broken heart or the delight of a heart filled with joy. The upper *dan tian* is situated in your head and is the source of your spiritual energy.

When practising tai chi, being aware of the vital points and energy fields can help make you more sensitive to changes in physical sensation in your body. You can stimulate your vital points by applying gentle pressure and massaging them, or by simply focusing on them.

In many ways, becoming aware of your energy fields simply involves redefining what you already experience. Most people habitually ignore, or at least fail to take seriously, the signals that their bodies give them. However, it is relatively easy to learn to listen to your body and to become aware of the physiological effect of

your emotions. For example, if you sit cooped up in an office all day and then go for a walk in a park, you may notice that you feel uplifted emotionally, that you feel better physically, or that you feel somehow energized. You could also say that your qi, or life energy, is stimulated.

ALIGNING AND EXPANDING QI

Try this simple exercise, evocatively named "aligning the Three Treasures: the Heavens, Earth, and Human", or "merging the light of heaven with the forms of the earth". It involves moving your awareness through each of the vital points and energy fields (*see opposite*). Think of the three points as entry points into the energy fields. These points are a common focus in tai chi because they are located at your extremities; concentrating on them can help establish a sense of connection with your entire body.

Find a quiet position outside, and stand upright with feet hip-width apart, arms by your sides, and your body relaxed and aligned. Concentrate on your breathing.
• **Focus on the Heavens:** sense the crown point and the upper *dan tian*; elevate your mind, and think beyond your immediate surroundings to the sun, sky, and stars. Be aware of your spiritual energy.
• **Focus on Earth:** notice the Bubbling Spring point and the lower *dan tian*; picture nature: water, soil, plants, flowers, and the physical world that surrounds you. Be aware of your physical connection to the world.
• **Focus on Human:** bring your attention to the Work Palace point and the middle *dan tian*; consider your personal energy and your connection to all life.

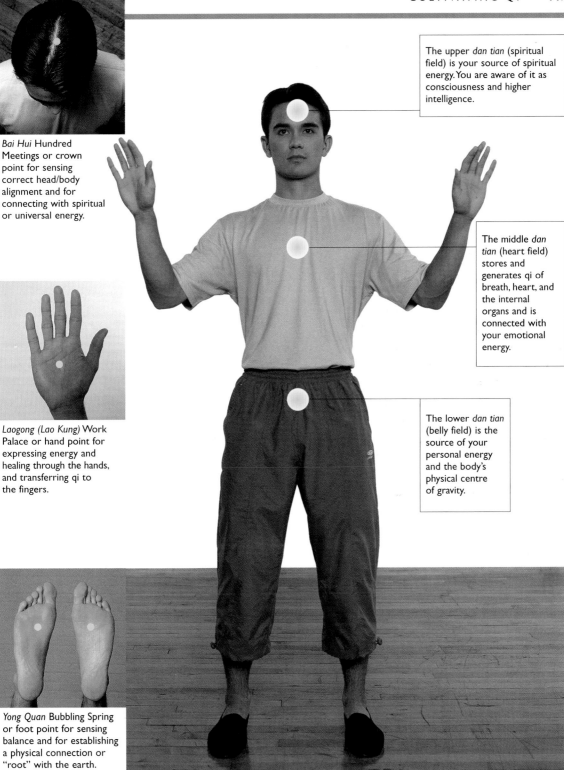

The upper *dan tian* (spiritual field) is your source of spiritual energy. You are aware of it as consciousness and higher intelligence.

Bai Hui Hundred Meetings or crown point for sensing correct head/body alignment and for connecting with spiritual or universal energy.

The middle *dan tian* (heart field) stores and generates qi of breath, heart, and the internal organs and is connected with your emotional energy.

Laogong (Lao Kung) Work Palace or hand point for expressing energy and healing through the hands, and transferring qi to the fingers.

The lower *dan tian* (belly field) is the source of your personal energy and the body's physical centre of gravity.

Yong Quan Bubbling Spring or foot point for sensing balance and for establishing a physical connection or "root" with the earth.

MOVING AND GATHERING QI

The exercises shown here provide practice in combining breathing with movement and mental focus. They help to relax you and to promote the flow of qi within the body. Practise as a sequence or individually either before or after a tai chi session. Remember to move slowly.

BREATHING CRANE

This qigong exercise moves energy between the lower and middle energy fields. It promotes emotional balance and can enhance overall physical vitality, or *jing*. Visualize the ball in this exercise as a ball of energy. Keep your shoulders and wrists relaxed. Practise this as a flowing sequence, or pause for a moment in each position.

2 As you begin to exhale, move your palms to face down at your solar plexus, as if resting on the top of the ball. Take care to keep your wrists relaxed and straight.

1 Stand in the *Horse Stance* with your hands at your belly, fingers facing each other as if holding a ball. Sense your feet and crown points. Breathe slowly and deeply. Sense your fingers and the vital points in your hands. Focus on your belly. Then inhale and bend your elbows to raise your hands to your solar plexus. As you do this, move your focus from the lower energy field (your belly) to the middle energy field (your heart).

3 As you continue to exhale, lower your hands towards your belly. As you do this, move your focus from the middle to the lower energy field. Repeat the entire movement 5 times or more, then pause for several breaths with your hands facing your belly.

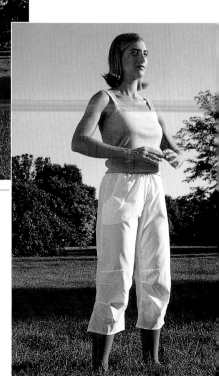

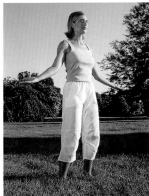

BATHING IN THE LIGHT

Light is the purest form of energy and is associated with the upper energy field and the crown point (*see p147*). Focus on breathing slowly and deeply, and contemplate the cleansing and healing properties of light as you gather qi in this exercise. Move in a flowing sequence, or pause for a few moments in each position.

1 Stand in the *Horse Stance* with your arms out to the sides, palms facing up and out. Breathe slowly and deeply. Sense the vital points in your feet, hands, and head. Visualize light surrounding your head, arms, and hands.

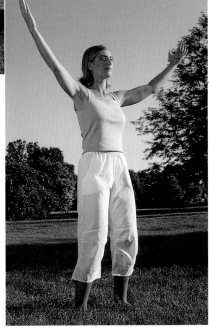

2 As you begin to inhale, raise your arms towards the sky so that your fingers point up and out. Feel into the tips of your fingers, and imagine that you are raising the light and holding it between your hands.

4 As you exhale, lower your hands in front of you, palms down, with the tips of your fingers pointing towards each other. Imagine that you are drawing the light down into your body and through your legs and feet. Repeat 5 times or more, then pause for several breaths.

3 As you continue to inhale, bend your elbows, bringing your fingers towards each other above your head. Imagine that they are resting on the light gathered above your head. Be aware of a connection between the vital points in your hands and the crown point.

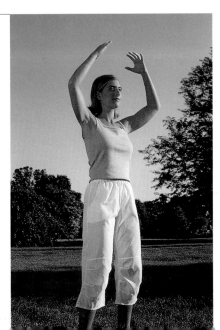

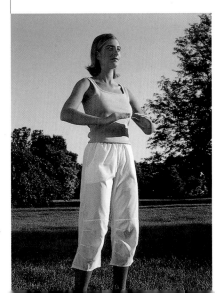

CONNECTING QI WITH A PARTNER

These exercises build skill in sensing qi with a partner. This ability is central to the martial arts application of tai chi: to remain peaceful and aware of your own energy while experiencing another person's energy in any situation, whether cooperative or hostile. Practise with someone with whom you feel comfortable, and avoid looking into your partner's eyes as this can be distracting. You may notice increased warmth, heaviness, or tingling in your hands, or a magnetic sensation. These are indications that you are sensing energy on a subtle level.

ATTUNING TO QI

Remain centred, rooted, and aligned during this exercise. You can practise the first position on your own to regulate personal qi. Hold each position for at least one minute. Remember to breathe deeply and slowly.

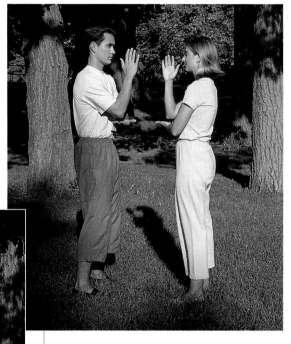

1 Stand facing each other in the *Horse Stance*. Each person positions their left hand under their own right elbow, right thumb pointing between their nose and mouth. Feel the sensation within your body. Move your left palm slightly to experience a change in sensation.

2 Move your left hand so your palm is under your partner's right elbow. Your partner does the same. Feel any changes in sensation within your body. Move your left palm slightly to experience changes in sensation. Finally, relax with your hands by your sides.

MOVING THE ENERGY BALL

This exercise helps you to coordinate breathing, movement, and mental focus with a partner. Practise it to experience both the receptive and active (yin and yang) elements of the *Push Position* in tai chi. Notice the increased energy when you move qi with your partner. Hold these positions for one minute or longer.

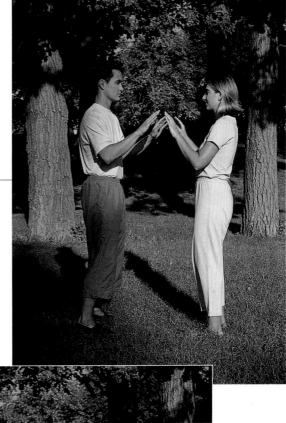

1 Stand facing each other in the *Horse Stance*, with hands in the tai chi *Push Position* — arms parallel, wrists relaxed, and palms facing forwards and slightly down. Focus on your own breathing, and notice the sensation in your palms and fingers. Coordinate your breathing so you both inhale and exhale at the same time.

2 As you inhale, bend your elbows and draw your hands away from each other in the *Push Position*. As you exhale, bring your hands closer together as in step 1. Repeat this 5 or more times, focusing on your breathing and on any changes in sensation in your hands. Practise moving your hands into different positions, maintaining this sense of connection. Finally, relax with your hands by your sides.

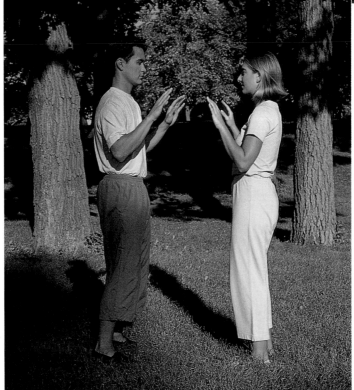

QI IN A GROUP

The sense of peacefulness that comes from practising tai chi in a group is like no other; it is a unique experience. Each person is centred within him- or herself, and at the same time extends this sense of connection to include all the others in the group. Staying in tune with your own body as you also feel the energy of the group will help you to strengthen your personal qi and expand your awareness of it.

After practising tai chi in a group, conclude the session by forming the qi circle. You need at least three people. Remain centred, rooted, and aligned, since this enhances your own energy and that of the circle. Ideally, practise this exercise outdoors in a peaceful setting.

THE QI CIRCLE

Stand in a circle with your arms relaxed, elbows heavy, and wrists relaxed and straight. Position your hands so that they face into the circle but are also angled towards the person on either side of you. Focus on slow, relaxed breathing and on your alignment. Take a few moments to centre and to sense each of your vital points and energy fields (*see pp146–147*).

Focus on any changes of sensation in your hands. Notice physical sensations in your body, and at the same time be aware of the larger group. Contemplate the symbolic significance of the circle — it has no beginning and no end. Similarly, tai chi, the Supreme Ultimate, encompasses all opposites, it is circular. Consider the tai chi symbol and the balance of yin and yang. Hold the position for 1–3 minutes or more.

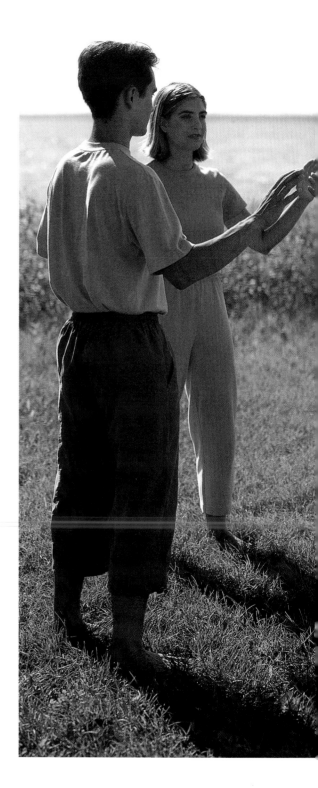

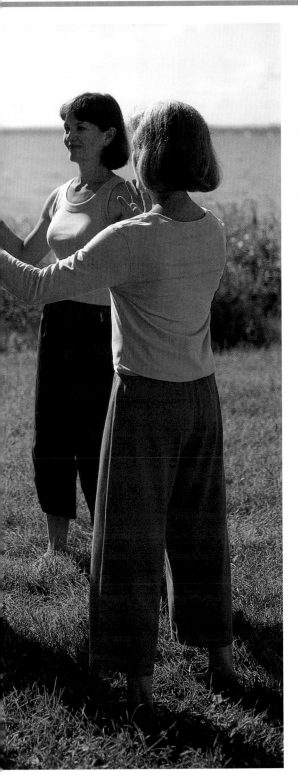

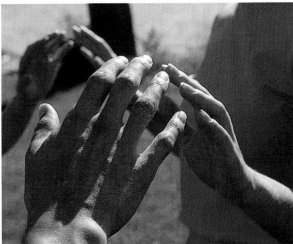

Your fingers are aligned with your neighbours' fingers, but do not touch. Focus on your hands and fingers, and notice any changes in sensation. Imagine a beam of light connecting the hand points around the circle.

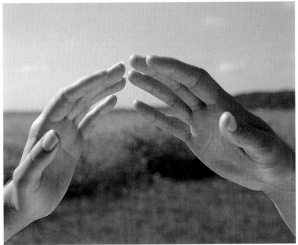

Hands are angled so that they partially face your neighbours' hands and also partially face towards the centre of the circle. This allows your shoulders and wrists to relax. Note that your hands do not directly face your neighbours' as they do when connecting qi with a partner.

GLOSSARY

Note: There are variations in Chinese spelling depending upon which transliteration system you use: the older Wade-Giles or the modern Pinyin. In this book, I have borrowed from both systems, using whatever spelling is most commonly recognized in English. So, for example, I chose the older, more familiar spelling of tai chi but the newer Pinyin spelling of qi because recently that has become more familiar to Westerners. Alternative spellings are shown in brackets after each entry.

Bai Hui (Bai Hwei)

(pronounced bye way): Hundred Channels or Hundred Meetings Point. Sensing this point helps you to position your head in correct alignment with your body, and to connect with and absorb spiritual or universal energy. Located at the crown of the head, it is an acupuncture point connecting the Governor and Conception Channels, the body's primary *yin* and *yang* channels.

Dan Tian (Tan T'ien)

(pronounced don tien): Vital Energy Field or Elixir Field, literally "cinnabar" or "red field". A reservoir for storing and generating the body's subtle energy. In *tai chi*, reference to the *dan tian* usually refers to the lower *dan tian*, however, there are three:
Lower *Dan Tian*: personal energy field. The lower *dan tian* is located in the belly, the body's physical centre of gravity. It is our primary field that stores and generates the *qi* of our physical body.
Middle *Dan Tian*: heart energy field. Located in the chest, it stores and generates *qi* of the breath, heart, and internal organs. In Chinese, the word for "mind", *hsin*, also means, "heart".
Upper *Dan Tian*: spiritual energy field. Located in the head, it stores *shen*, or spirit, consciousness, and higher intelligence.

Jing (Ching)

(pronounced jing): Physical or sexual energy. It is considered to be a *yin* or earthy form of *qi*.

Kwa (Gua)

(pronounced gwa): The hip joint; specifically, the place where the hip joint forms a crease at the top of the femur or thighbone. It is a key area of focus when practising the Tai Chi Fold.

Laogong (Lao Kung)

(pronounced low gung): Work Palace or Labour Temple. Located in the centre of the palms, this point is for expressing energy and healing through the hands, and transferring *qi* to the fingers. Its meridian connects with the heart. It is an acupuncture point on the pericardium meridian. (The pericardium is the protective sac that surrounds the heart; it is considered a separate organ in Chinese medicine.)

Qi (Ch'i or Chi)

(pronounced chee): Vital energy or life force, the energy that permeates all living things. It is a commonly used term in everyday Chinese language. For example, weather is *tien qi* or heaven energy, air is *kung qi* or empty energy, air conditioner is lung *qi ji* or cold energy machine, anger is *sheng qi* or energy rising.

Qigong (Ch'i Kung)

(pronounced chee gung): Vital energy cultivation. This term refers to a variety of moving, standing, and sitting exercises that promote the flow of *qi* in the body. *Tai chi* is a form of *qigong*.

Shen

(pronounced shen): Spiritual energy or spirit. It is considered to be a yang or universal form of *qi*.

Sung

(pronounced soong): Active relaxation. This term also means "to sink". It is a state of being calm, alert, and energetic.

Tai Chi (Taiji)

(pronounced tai chee): Supreme ultimate. The unifying still point, the Grand Terminus or Ridge Post that connects the heavens and earth. The *ying–yang* symbol is called the *tai chi* diagram in Chinese.

Tai Chi Ch'uan (Taijiquan)

(pronounced tai chee chew-an): Supreme ultimate boxing. *Tai chi* means "the unifying still point, the Grand Terminus or Ridge Post connecting the heavens and earth". Ch'uan or Quan means "boxing" or "fist".

Tao (Dao)

(pronounced dow): Path or road that is in harmony with the larger universe, the natural world, and oneself. Also referred to as the "middle way", the "way of nature", and "the path of peace".

Wu Chi (Wuji)

(pronounced wu jee): Undivided unity, or primordial state of infinite potential in the universe that gives birth to *yin* and *yang* polarity. It is represented as the outer circle in the *tai chi* or *yin–yang* symbol.

Yin and Yang

The two distinctive expressions of *Wu Chi* or unity that give rise to countless variations. *Yin* is cool, dark, passive, earth; *Yang* represents hot, bright, active, sky.

Yong Ch'uan (Yong Quan)

(pronounced yung chew-an): Bubbling Well or Bubbling Spring Point for sensing balance and for establishing "root". It is located at the centre of the foot, just below the ball. Focus on this point to "ground" yourself when experiencing fear. It is an acupuncture point on the kidney meridian; stimulating it helps to clam you down and also lowers blood pressure.

RESOURCES

Tai chi classes are often taught through the following organizations: health clubs and gyms, sports and leisure centres, adult education institutes, community centres, universities and colleges, and specialist clubs. Tai chi schools may be listed under the following headings in your telephone book: Martial Arts, Sports Clubs and Associations, and Sports Training and Coaching. Check your local health food store and alternative bookseller for posters advertising classes.

USEFUL CONTACTS
Willam C.C. Chen
Tai Chi Ch'uan
12 West 23rd Street, 2nd fl.
New York, New York 10010
USA
Tel: (212) 675–2816
www.williamccchen.com
Grandmaster, author; conducts workshops worldwide.

Ken Cohen
Qigong Research and
Practice Center
PO Box 1727
Nederland, Colorado 80466
USA
Tel: (303) 258–0971
www.qigonghealing.com
Qigong master, author; conducts workshops worldwide.

Welstone: Laura Stone and
Fred van Welsem
T.G. Gibsonstraat 33
7411 RP Deventer
The Netherlands
Tel: 011 31 570–615305
www.welstone.nl
Applied Tai–Chi Ch'uan, conflict resolution training, mediation.

Tai Chi Union for Great Britain
1 Littlemill Drive
Balmoral Gardens
Crookston
Glasgow G53 7GF
Tel: 0141–810–3482
Email: secretary@taichiunion.com
www.taichiunion.com
Includes a national list of over 350 registered instructors. Produces a twice yearly magazine, Tai Chi Chuan.

The British Council for Chinese
Martial Arts
c/o 110 Frensham Drive
Stockingford
Warwickshire CV10 9QL
Email: infor@bccma.demon.co.uk
www.bccma.org.uk
The official governing body for Chinese Martial Arts in the UK. Provides details of local tai chi classes.

Vicki A. Wood
Upper Curragh
Feakle
County Clare
Ireland
Tel: 00 353 (0) 61–924974
Email: ellenderj@eircom.net

OTHER USEFUL WEBSITES
www.taichifinder.co.uk
Tai chi finder in the UK and Ireland. Includes information on tai chi videos, reading material, and equipment, in addition to listing class schedules all over the UK.

www.taichichuan.co.uk
Practical Tai–Chi Ch'uan online. Offers a wealth of information on UK classes and the history, background and philosophy of tai chi.

www.dongtaichi.com/london
Dong Family International Tai–Chi Ch'uan Association. Useful website that gives general information on tai chi; lists classes in London for all levels.

TAI CHI MAGAZINES
Tai Chi Magazine
PO Box 39938
Los Angeles, California 90039
USA
Tel: (323) 665–7773
www.tai-chi.com
The leading international magazine of tai chi.

Tai Chi Chuan
Published by the Tai Chi Union for Great Britain.

Qi Magazine
Tse Qigong Centre
PO Box 59
Altrincham WA15 8FS
Tel: 0161–929–4485
Email: tse@qimagazine.com

FURTHER READING

Chen, William, *Body Mechanics of T'ai–Chi Ch'uan*
Wm. CC Chen, 2 Washington Square Village #10J, New York, NY 10012; 8th edition, 1999.

Cohen, Kenneth, *The Way of Qigong*
Ballantine Books, New York, NY; 1997.

Chopra, Deepak, *Ageless Body Timeless Mind*
Harmony Books, New York, NY; 1993.

Gia Fu Feng, *Tao Te Ching*
Random House, New York, NY; 1972.

Garripoli, Garri, *Qigong: Essence of the Healing Dance*
Health Communications, Inc.; 1999.

Lo, Benjamin and Inn, Martin (Translators), *Cheng Tzu's Thirteen Treaties on T'ai–Chi Ch'uan*
North Atlantic Books, Berkeley, CA; 1985.

Lo, Benjamin et al (Translators), *The Essence of T'ai–Chi Ch'uan*
North Atlantic Books, Berkeley, CA; 1985.

Lowenthal, Wolfe, *There Are No Secrets: Professor Cheng Man Ch'ing and His T'ai–Chi Ch'uan*
North Atlantic Books, Berkeley, CA; 1991.

Man-Ching Cheng and Smith, Robert, *Tai–Chi*
Tuttle, VT; 1967.

Mitchell, Stephen, *Tao Te Ching*
Harper and Rowe, New York, NY; 1988.

Tsung Hwa Jou, *The Dao of Taijiquan*
T'ai-Chi Foundation, Tuttle, VT; 1988.

Ueshiba, Morihei and Stevens, John (Translator), *The Art of Peace*
Shambala, Boston, MA; 1992.

Wile, Douglas, *Master Cheng's Thirteen Chapters on T'ai–Chi Ch'uan*
Sweet Chi Press, New York, NY; 1982.

Tricia Yu has produced several DVDs and videos that make useful accompaniments to this book:

Tai Chi Fundamentals for Mastering Tai Chi Basics
DVD and video
Instruction in the Basic Moves and Form taught in this book.

Tai Chi Fundamentals: Training for Health Care Professionals and Instructors
video and manual
Instruction in the Basic Moves and Form taught in this book. Includes clinical analysis and therapeutic benefits of the Basic Moves.

Energize: Daily Warm–Ups for Flexibility and Strength
video
Instruction in a complete stretching and strengthening routine that includes all warm-ups featured in this book.

Tai Chi: Exercise for Lifelong Health and Well–Being
DVD and video
Instruction in the Yang-Style Short Form, Chen Man-Ching Lineage.

For further informaton, or to purchase videos and DVDs, contact:
Uncharted Country Publishing
www.taichihealth.com
Tel: 1 800–488–4940
Tel: (608) 280–9730
Fax: (608) 280–9736
Email: ucp@taichihealth.com

Available in the UK from
Quantum Leap
www.qleap.co.uk
Tai Chi Fundamentals Video and DVD; Ynag Style Cheng Man Ching Lineage Form Video

TO CONTACT TRICIA YU
The Tai Chi Center
301 South Bedford Street
Madison
Wisconsin 53703
Tel: (608) 257–4171
Email: tcc@taichihealth.com

INDEX

ACKNOWLEDGMENTS

AUTHOR'S ACKNOWLEDGMENTS

Although I am listed as sole author, this book is presented to you thanks to drudgery and jolly times with DK's fantastic team of experts. Profound gratitude to Nasim Mawji for her patience, unfailing sense of humour, and remarkable skill at making things clear, concise, and sensible. Thanks to Tracy Killick, for her bravado and brilliance and, with Graham Atkins-Hughes, for their collaborative genius in expressing both form and essence on film. To dear Jenny Jones for embracing and seeing this project through, and to Mary-Clare Jerram for her guidance and support. Thanks also to Gillian Roberts, Nick Rayment, Mary Nahn, Nathan McQuillen, and Bill Mason. Special thanks to the models Sara Tripalin, Kai Yu, and Patricia Culotti for their dedication and good cheer.

Deep appreciation to those who have helped along the path. In chronological order: a lifetime of gratitude to my parents, Robert and Mildred Beadles, for the foundation of unconditional love, and to Robert Lin-I Yu who opened the doorway to the East. To Taoist Master Liu Pei Ch'ung, Tai Chi Masters Benjamin Pang Jeng Lo, William C.C. Chen, and Maggie Newman, and to Paul Gallagher, Wei Mo Zhu, and Li Jun Feng for guidance and inspiration. Thanks to colleagues Diane Harlowe, Jill Johnson, and Betty Chewning for our collaborations in bringing tai chi into therapeutic and fitness circles. Thanks to tai chi sisters Patricia Culotti and Lauri Mckean for sharing the journey. Special thanks to Eva Wright, Carol Karls, Judy Smith, Gail Janz, Sarah Caroll, Kimberly Stillman, and Jessica Athens. Most of all to my beloved husband, Douglas Swayne, for making sure that we paddle with both oars in the water.

PUBLISHER'S ACKNOWLEDGMENTS

Dorling Kindersley would like to thank photographer Graham Atkins-Hughes and his assistant, Nick Rament; Mary Nahn of Blush Productions for hair and make-up, Liz Hancock for clothes styling. Thank you to Rubin's furniture store, Olbrich Botanical Gardens, Monona Terrace, and the City of Madison Parks Department for shoot locations. Thanks to the models: Sara, Kai, and Pat, and to the cover model, Alison Smith.

PHOTOGRAPHIC ACKNOWLEDGMENTS

Specially commissioned photography by Graham Atkins-Hughes at A and R Associates. The publisher would like to thank the following for their kind permission to reproduce their photographs: 9: Henry A. Koshollek; 14: Mike de Vries.
All other images © Dorling Kindersley.
For further information see www.dkimages.com

ABOUT THE AUTHOR

Tricia Yu, MA, is the owner and director of the Tai Chi Centre in Madison, Wisconsin, one of the oldest and largest schools in the United States. She has taught tai chi, qigong, and meditation since 1972, introducing tai chi to thousands of people through her classes, public presentations, and professional training seminars. Her teaching has always emphasized the health of body, mind, and spirit. Tricia has devised programmes that make tai chi accessible to people with a wide range of abilities and she was the first to integrate tai chi into medical exercise therapy. Tricia began her study of tai chi in the Republic of China in 1970 with Master Liu Pei Ch'ung. She studies with Tai Chi Master Benjamin Pang Jeng Lo, Maggie Newman, and Grandmaster William C.C. Chen. She is certified by Grandmaster Chen.